ULTRA-PROCESSED WOMEN

ULTRA-PROCESSED WOMEN

Milli Hill

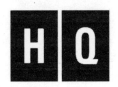

ONE PLACE. MANY STORIES

HQ
An imprint of HarperCollins*Publishers* Ltd
1 London Bridge Street
London SE1 9GF

www.harpercollins.co.uk

HarperCollins*Publishers*
Macken House, 39/40 Mayor Street Upper,
Dublin 1, D01 C9W8, Ireland

This edition 2025

1
First published in Great Britain by
HQ, an imprint of HarperCollins*Publishers* Ltd 2025

Copyright © Milli Hill 2025

Milli Hill asserts the moral right to be identified as the author of this work.
A catalogue record for this book is available from the British Library.

HB ISBN: 978-0-00-872180-0
TPB ISBN: 978-0-00-872179-4

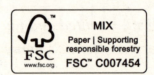

This book contains FSC™ certified paper and other controlled
sources to ensure responsible forest management.

For more information visit: www.harpercollins.co.uk/green

This book is set in 10.7/15.5 pt. Sabon by Type-it AS, Norway

Printed and Bound in the UK using 100% Renewable Electricity at
CPI Group (UK) Ltd, Croydon, CR0 4YY

All rights reserved. No part of this publication may be reproduced, stored in a retrieval system, or transmitted, in any form or by any means, electronic, mechanical, photocopying, recording or otherwise, without the prior permission of the publishers.

Without limiting the author's and publisher's exclusive rights, any unauthorised use of this publication to train generative artificial intelligence (AI) technologies is expressly prohibited. HarperCollins also exercise their rights under Article 4(3) of the Digital Single Market Directive 2019/790 and expressly reserve this publication from the text and data mining exception.

This book is dedicated to my own personal celestial trinity:

Gilbert Hill 1926–2014
Bert Back 1922–2000
Paul Barrett 1944–2022

I like to think of them, reunited and raising a glass to this book, in one of the afterlife's many perfect pubs.

Contents

Introduction *But what about women?*   1

1. **So, what is ultra-processed food (UPF)?**
   And is it even food at all?   15

2. **What's the problem with UPF?**
   And why are we suddenly talking about it now?   37

3. **A woman's place**
   The kitchen and promises of liberation   59

4. **Start them young**
   How the UPF industry exploits mothers and children   75

5. **Ben? Jerry? I'm breaking up with you!**
   Obesity and women's toxic relationship with UPF   97

6. **An apple a day keeps the OBGYN away**
   The care and feeding of your female microbiome   117

7. **Unlucky women?**
   Are we too accepting of women's suffering?   139

8. **I'll have the blues**
   Depression on the menu   163

9. **Ageing like fine cheese**
   UPF in the second half of life   185

10. **A delicious tub of face cream**
    The disturbing overlaps of UPF and cosmetics   211

11. **Disrespecting the Mother**
    How UPF damages the Earth   229

12. **Seeds of change**
    How to quit or reduce UPF   253

Postscript: *A dog's dinner*   303
Acknowledgements   309
Resources   311
Endnotes   317
Index   371

Introduction

But what about women?

When I first began work on this book, I thought it was going to be about food. Oh, and women, of course – I nearly forgot – it's funny how often that happens, isn't it? We forget women. So yes, food – and women: this was to be my focus. I'd noticed some really interesting conversations beginning about what we, as twenty-first-century humans, are eating and what this might be doing to our bodies. I'd also noticed that such discussions were almost always generalized in terms of the possible negative impact on 'people's' health. Male 'people' are different in a variety of ways from female 'people', but this simple fact is still repeatedly overlooked and, worse still, male people can be treated as the default or prototype human. So I found myself listening with interest to the many discussions about 'ultra-processed food' (UPF) and wondering to myself: 'But what about women?'

But what about women?

If ever there was a question that slips out of the collective consciousness far too readily, it's that one. If you are in a position of power or influence, consider jotting it at the top of your notebook page, or setting it as your screensaver, or perhaps getting it as a tattoo. It's not asked nearly as often as it should be, and as the conversation buzzed about the hot topic of UPF, it seemed to be missing yet again. *But what about women?* As a writer on women's health, and also as a busy mum of three who spends a great deal of time preoccupied with the thorny issue of 'what's for dinner?', I decided to try to answer it myself.

Setting out to investigate, much of my initial focus was on the female body, and the possible impact of our modern, ultra-processed diet on our physical health. In telling people about this book, I've discovered that this is often their assumption about the subject matter, too. 'I'm writing a book about ultra-processed food and the impact on women,' I say. 'Oh... like menopause and stuff?', they reply. And yes, it's true that some of this book explores the possible detrimental impact of a diet high in UPF on women's reproductive health: menstrual cycles, gynaecological health issues, fertility, pregnancy and, yes, menopause. Much of what I have found in the existing research has shocked me and reinforced yet again just how readily we accept the idea of the female body as naturally faulty and in need of medicalization – these assumptions often blinding us to other potential, and often less invasive, courses of action. Obviously we don't want to turn our backs on modern medicine's often very helpful input, but it would be great if we could shift towards a more holistic approach. Imagine what might change if the question, 'what do you eat?', was top of the list for any woman struggling with some aspect of her reproductive health? How many women suffering painful or heavy periods, for example, might be interested to know that

INTRODUCTION

reducing the amount of UPF they consume and eating fruits and pulses instead might be a game-changer? How many pregnant women, fastidiously avoiding pâté or blue cheese, might wonder why nobody told them that a diet high in UPF could potentially double their risk of miscarriage, or that fizzy drinks had been associated with a raft of pregnancy issues from pre-term birth to health problems like asthma in their baby? Why isn't every single couple struggling with the agony of infertility being told that a move away from UPF and towards a more Mediterranean-style diet could have a positive impact on both female fertility and male sperm count? And – regardless of whether or not women in perimenopause choose to take HRT – shouldn't they all know that replacing the UPF in their diet with healthier choices, like wholefoods and plants, could reduce their symptoms by as much as 34 per cent?[1]

Periods, fertility, pregnancy, menopause – these are all hugely important to women's health and can have a massive impact on our entire life story. But women are not walking wombs, and to answer the question *'but what about women?'* by simply focusing on the various activities of our uterus would be to continue the centuries-long habit of reducing us down to our reproductive potential. It would also risk leaving you aside if you are reading this book as a younger woman who isn't particularly concerned with having kids, or indeed, an older woman who is child-free. There are many other areas of health – depression, autoimmune conditions, obesity, disordered eating and more – where ensuring women are front and centre in both discussion and research about the impact of UPF is vital. Women are twice as likely to suffer from depression as men, and researchers have repeatedly found that UPF could be increasing our risk: in one study by as much as 50 per cent;[2] in another, which studied those who already had depressive symptoms, support to change diet away from UPF led to one-third of participants meeting the criteria for remission.[3] Similarly, autoimmune conditions, which also disproportionately affect women, are increasingly being found to be impacted by diet: lupus, for example, affects nine times as many women as men, and recent research has found that women consuming the highest amounts of UPF are over 50 per cent more likely to develop it.[4] For so many women, ending their toxic relationship with UPF is potentially life-changing.

As we wake up to the impact of UPF on our health, it's important to remember that there are billion-dollar global corporations whose revenue is at stake if we all start having an egg salad for lunch washed down with a glass of water. And they are not going to go quietly. As we learn to flip the packets over and read labels, those labels are going to change. There is even a phrase for this in the food industry: 'clean labelling'. In some cases, this may be a genuine effort to reduce the number of additives and unnatural UPF ingredients in products; in other cases, it's a more cynical tactic to choose ingredients that appear more 'natural', for example 'rosemary extract', which sounds straight out of the herb garden, but is actually chemically extracted from the plant using solvents resulting in a brown, antioxidant powder. As the UPF conversation grows, it's also important to 'follow the money' – even dieticians, authors and influencers with the best intentions may have their views swayed by free trips to conferences sponsored by food companies. Chris van Tulleken, who has moved the conversation so far forward with his book *Ultra-Processed People*, has reported being offered £20,000 to give a talk for a food company. The deal involved signing a contract to never disparage their brand, 'through the universe and in perpetuity'. He declined, and describes the influence of Big Food as 'tentacular'.

Analysis from the *British Medical Journal* in 2024 revealed these tentacles reach into the corridors of power, and that more than half of the experts on the UK government's advisory panel on nutrition have links to the UK food industry.[5] One paper that was published while I was writing this book states that there isn't enough evidence about the obesity risk of UPF, and that avoiding this type of food could even be *risky* – but a closer look reveals one of the authors is on the scientific advisory board for the confectionary multinational Mars.[6] And in Australia, experts have warned that UPF companies are exerting too much influence over food labelling, exploiting the focus on nutrient content terms like 'low fat' or 'high protein' and allowing some foods to be labelled as healthy choices when they are anything but.[7] Whoever is advising you about UPF, from your favourite Instagram foodie to your government, don't forget that nobody is above influence in our current ultra-processed world.

As my work on this book deepened, I began to see that, even beyond these important topics of health research and influence, there is still much more to discuss. As I listened to podcasts and read books and articles about UPF, and began to try to implement change in my own family life, I started noticing a response in myself that was more emotional than physical, and it felt all too familiar: mum-guilt. If you're not already aware, mum-guilt is that feeling so many of us get when a standard is set and we are unable to meet it. Whether it's a parenting choice, an immaculate home, or just a sense that we should be enjoying our time with our children more than we actually are, the possibilities for mum-guilt are absolutely endless, and only made worse by social media giving us immediate access to other women seemingly breezing through their days in a state of bouncy fulfilment. We watch their reels about how to fit in your yoga practice around home-schooling your kids and running your own PR agency and *wham!*: mum-guilt, there it is. Rooted in the deep and powerful love we have for our children and our sense of inadequacy, failure and anxiety when we feel we are not doing our absolute best for them, mum-guilt seems to be consistently the preserve of women. And as I pushed my trolley round the supermarket and tried to contemplate life without UPF, here was mum-guilt again, winking at me from the freezer section and saying, 'why can't you make your own hash browns, it's easy-peasy!' All the books and podcasts were telling me that UPF was a problem that 'people' were going to have to solve, but again I wondered, 'what about women?' Was this UPF thing going to be yet another weight that women were going to have to add to their mental load, yet another bar set impossibly high, yet another area of life to be constantly worrying about, frequently failing at, and forever feeling guilty for?

If we tackle the topic of UPF, there's no point in pretending we've reached some kind of utopia where men and women take

INTRODUCTION

equal responsibility in the home for shopping, meal planning and food preparation. We need to acknowledge that there are wonderfully diverse families out there, as well as many good men who can make a mean tagliatelle, but that in a lot of homes it's women who do the lion's share of the cooking. This is particularly true of homes with young children, but it can even apply in the case of shared flats of young students or friends. Worldwide, on average, women cook twice as many meals as men.[8] It's important to be aware of the potential burden that may fall on women if we start saying everyone should be cooking their food from scratch, but at the same time it's interesting to flip this question on its head and ask: why have we all absorbed this idea that cooking and food preparation is 'drudgery' – menial work that's a complete waste of time compared to important stuff like *actual* 'work'? Is it really feminist progress to heat up a microwave meal after a long day at the office, or is this just a lie we've been sold by food companies, keen to line their pockets by convincing us that cooking, like so many other traditional female roles – cleaning, teaching, nursing, caring – is low value and should be outsourced whenever possible?

I write this book as someone who likes cooking and eating, but who also sometimes wishes that being an adult didn't require showing up each day with a plan for dinner. I am not a nutritionist, or doctor, or health guru; I have no diet product or supplement to sell; and so far I've not been approached by any food companies with a fat cheque and an all-inclusive trip to Italy. Nor am I a 'perfect mum' who has raised her kids on sourdough and homemade granola. I'm basically just another woman looking around at the world we've all created and wondering, is this the best we can do? Is this freedom? As a Gen X'er, I was a little girl in the 1980s and grew up with the idea of 'having it all'. Ambition, and even greed, was a good thing, according to Michael Douglas's character in the 1987 movie *Wall Street* anyway. Working nine to five and hopefully having a glittering career that involved shoulder pads wasn't just a choice, it was an obligation. We scoffed at our school lessons in cookery and sewing, both referred to as 'Home Economics', and thought of them as archaic throwbacks to a terrible era of female imprisonment that would thankfully never apply to us. But as 'having it all' played out its course, many of us, particularly the ones hit by the motherhood juggernaut, have wondered through gritted teeth if the whole concept might need a bit of a tweak. In spite of the promises of convenience and liberation, my generation of women – and the next few gens after me – seem more knackered than ever, expected to 'work like we don't have children and raise children like we don't work', constantly under pressure to curate perfect Insta-worthy homes, perfect childhoods for our kids, perfect ageless faces, perfect toned abs, all while building some kind of career portfolio. So believe me when I say, this book is not intending to add to that to-do list. By centring women in the UPF conversation, this book is not here to put them in charge of solving the UPF problem, particularly not if this means remembering to put mung beans on to soak at 11 p.m.

What this book does want to do is to ask: what do we all really want? Because as I've gone deeper and deeper into the

INTRODUCTION

topic of UPF, I've come to see that the contents of our store cupboards, trolleys and dinner plates are not really about food at all – they're a reflection of the values of our current culture and, ultimately, a sign of our direction of travel as a species. There are running themes when we begin to think about UPF that we can find elsewhere in our lives: mindless consumption; quantity over quality; lack of human contact; disconnection from nature; never having enough time. As we peer at our phone screens rather than look our friends and families in the eye, we ourselves become ultra-processed. We dull our animal instincts and forget our deep need to be in nature. We lose our ability to focus or to stick with something slow-moving or challenging. We find it harder and harder to read books. We spend on average nearly five hours a day on our phones,[9] and yet – and I am as guilty of this as the next person – we say we don't have enough time. Scrolling through our 'feed' (ironic that it's called this, isn't it?) is starving us of time outdoors, shared activities with friends, lovemaking, gardening, hugs, fitness and, yes, cooking and eating together. The global pandemic, with its zoom meetings, lockdowns and face masks, has only exacerbated this growing collective social anxiety and disconnectedness. We all know that sitting on our butts, endlessly doomscrolling, is making us mentally and physically unwell. And yet we continue: swipe up, swipe up, swipe up; discarding and consuming and discarding again on a repetitive cycle.

Consume…discard. In the past, and in indigenous cultures even today, people have taken and continue to take a different approach to their food. Often this has been reflected in rituals that encourage mindfulness. 'For what we are about to receive, may the Lord make us truly thankful,' is one such example, and even those of us who, like me, are not religious, can perhaps see the value in pausing together to reflect and express gratitude before picking up their fork. In Scotland, hunters traditionally say the Gralloch prayer – 'Life given for life' – offering thanks to the animal before or shortly after it is killed, and this kind of 'slaughter ritual' can be found across many cultures. Even a few muttered words embed a sense of gratitude to the life being taken, and some, like the Cree people of northeastern Canada, believe that the animal is not 'taken' at all but offers itself to them in a spirit of love and goodwill, ensuring the Earth and its people continue. Expressions of gratitude are not just confined to meat, either – many Native American cultures make offerings to plants and ask their permission before harvesting, and 'harvest' itself is celebrated globally, from Thanksgiving, to Diwali, to that extra-large marrow you carried up to the church altar in your school Harvest Festival. These acknowledgements of the interconnectedness of life and our interdependence with nature are now almost entirely missing from the Western world, where our approach to food has become entirely thoughtless and exploitative. UPF disconnects us and our children from the process of food preparation: washing, peeling, chopping, the nature of each ingredient. Our meat, as well as most of our other food items, is wrapped in plastic and obtained as we push a trolley mindlessly round brightly lit supermarkets. In the UK alone, an estimated ten million tonnes of that food is then thrown away each year.[10]

INTRODUCTION

The 'weekly shop' and even the supermarket itself are both relatively modern concepts. The supermarket as we now know it has evolved slowly over the twentieth century, and with each incremental change we have lost a little more connection to both our food and to our fellow humans. Up until around the 1950s, for example, the idea of 'self-service' – literally helping yourself to things from the shelves – didn't really exist. If I squint hard into my own memories, I can still remember those 'corner shops' with counters, where a kindly lady in tabard apron would 'serve' you. In the 1980s, my grandad had a newsagents with a counter at the back where he would slice ham and cheese for customers. The cheese slice was a particular fascination of mine, a seemingly magical long wire with a handle at the end that he would pull taut and splice downwards through the cheese, and then individually wrap the required amount in greaseproof paper. Shopkeeping was a job of great pride; it meant knowing people's names and what they usually ordered, and remembering whether it was a knee operation or a son's new college place that needed to be asked after. But by the 1980s this way of doing things was rapidly becoming obsolete, and we now find ourselves not only picking up our plastic-wrapped food ourselves but also beeping it out in the self-service checkout, without speaking to anyone unless the computer announces we have an unexpected item in the bagging area. And even as I write, this is evolving into the latest concept – a checkout-free store, where AI enables us to choose our items and simply leave, with our payment taken automatically. That is, if we complete our shop in a physical space at all – around half of us now buy at least some of our groceries online, and 16 per cent order all or most of our food via the internet. All of these steps have dehumanized our shopping experience, removing our contact with the food itself and also, of course, with chatty people like Bert, my grandad.

Ideas about the 'good old days' or the values of indigenous cultures can sound a bit twee. Much of human progress is positive and some habits of our forebears – women chained to the kitchen sink whether they liked it or not, for example – are best left behind us in the dust. But the current focus on UPF highlights that, as a species, we have lost our way – and this has happened very recently. In terms of human history, people have only abandoned their deep connection to the food on their plate in the last handful of decades, and yet we are rapidly forgetting things we have always known. As you will see in chapter 1, in order to work out whether a food is UPF or not, it's necessary to read the ingredients on the back of the packet, but I want to encourage you to think beyond this, too, to the idea of food being something we honour and respect. We are what we eat, but we also eat what we are. And, at the moment, we are ultra-processed; mindless consumers and discarders who have forgotten our connections to nature, to our food, and to each other. Look at the contents of your trolley or the food on your plate this evening. What story does it tell about you, and about this fleetingly brief moment in the many millennia of humans sitting down to eat?

And what about women? In the past few decades we've been encouraged to see everything from jam to baking to home-cooked family meals as an antiquated, anti-feminist waste of time. But perhaps we need reminding that it was never cooking or the kitchen that was holding us back from our freedom, it was the system of patriarchy. Now that, in the Western world at least, we have made some progress towards equality, maybe it's time to reconsider our relationship with food. Perhaps there is something to reclaim here; perhaps food offers us a way back to the interpersonal connection and mindfulness that we all acknowledge is rapidly slipping through humanity's fingers?

As women, we can instigate change. In a world where our human relationships and our health are both clearly at risk, lovingly preparing and eating a meal with others can be a revolutionary act. Sitting around a table of food has a similar effect to sitting around a campfire: it takes us back to our roots and it intuitively feels familiar, comforting and right. This simple act of shared humanity is also a valid act of resistance; a refusal to become ultra-processed women. In the UPF conversation, people often talk about 'quitting UPF' or 'giving it up'. But maybe we need to focus not on what we are giving up, but on what we are refusing to participate in, and also on what we might be bringing back or adding into our lives if we start eating real food again. So come with me as we explore ultra-processed food and its impact on females from every angle: from our weight to our microbes; from our fertility to our kids; from our emotions to our health in age; from the contents of our make-up bag to the impact on Mother Earth. But keep in the back of your mind that this is not just a book about food. Or women. (Let's not forget women.) It's about mindfulness, gratitude, love, connection, nature, and the very future of humanity.

1.

So, what is ultra-processed food (UPF)?

And is it even food at all?

Go into your nearest 7-Eleven or grocery store and just stand still for a moment. Look around. Notice the prepacked sandwiches, the yoghurts in plastic pots, the brightly coloured boxes of cereals, the microwave meals for one, the freezer pizzas, the doughnuts with their epic shelf-life. Now imagine yourself as a time-traveller. Maybe you've swung by via horse-and-carriage from Victorian England, or maybe Marty McFly picked you up this morning from your Stone Age settlement, or perhaps you're from somewhere else. It doesn't really matter where you imagine yourself having time-travelled from, because if you are human and from literally any period or place in the world prior to around 1970, you won't recognize any of this stuff at all. You will be unlikely to even identify it as food. Almost everything you see as you look around the shelves (even a small convenience store carries thousands of items, larger supermarkets may have tens of thousands) is very likely to be ultra-processed food (UPF). Of course, there are obvious exceptions. Most of us could work out that an apple or an egg – easily recognizable to our time-traveller – are not

UPF, but what about all that other stuff? How do you know what is UPF and what isn't?

Naming the problem

People have tried to define UPF in a variety of ways; for example, the food writer Michael Pollan has used the term 'edible foodlike substances', while doctor and author of *Ultra-Processed People*, Chris van Tulleken, explains it as anything 'wrapped in plastic and with at least one ingredient that you would not find in your kitchen'. Van Tulleken also suggests that another warning sign is packaging plastered with messages like, 'low fat', 'high in fibre' or 'supports your family's health' because almost every food with such health claims on the packet is UPF. Food writer Bee Wilson points out that UPFs are 'so altered that it can be hard to recognize the underlying ingredients', calling them 'concoctions of concoctions'. The current definition on Wikipedia describes them as 'industrially formulated edible substances'.

You'll notice that there's a distinct reluctance from all of these voices to refer to UPF as 'food' and, indeed, many argue that we should stop calling it this. Most recently, researchers at the Nova Institute for Health in Maryland have argued that the term 'food' is a misnomer and '...sits in foundational misalignment with how food has been defined, perceived, deliberated on, engaged with, and experienced by humans over millennia'. Rather than calling these 'hyper-palatable industrial items' food, they argue that they are so harmful and so far from nutrition that we should refer to them instead as UPP or 'ultra-processed products'.[1] For the purpose of clarity

SO, WHAT IS ULTRA-PROCESSED FOOD (UPF)?

in this book, I will continue to use UPF, but it's worth keeping in the back of your mind that many consider UPF to be undeserving of the word food at all.

If we wanted to put it really simply we could summarize UPF as 'factory-made food-like products' because, to be honest, there are not a great many foods that are made in a factory, packaged up and sitting on the supermarket shelf that wouldn't count as 'ultra-processed'. We could particularly point to food that has high numbers of ingredients that we do not recognize. We could begin to be vigilant about this notion of 'hyper-palatability' – food that we tend to keep eating even when we're full because it's just so moreish. And we could define UPF as 'food that's made for maximum profit' because UPF is not just industrially processed, it inevitably has added ingredients that are designed to bulk it up, make it last longer, make it look better, improve its texture, increase its profit margins and, above all, make you want to eat more of it than you truly need. UPF is food that puts the revenue of multinational food companies first, and your long-term health and nutrition last – if it considers that at all.

In summary, something is likely to be UPF if it ticks the following boxes:

- ingredients you don't recognize as food;
- made in a factory and packaged in branded, appealing plastic packaging with health claims;
- hyperpalatable, i.e. tasty and moreish;
- low-cost ingredients, heavily marketed, for maximum profit.

What's the difference between 'processed' and 'ultra-processed'?

People have always processed their food, at least for a very, very long time. Taking raw ingredients and doing things to them to make them tastier or longer lasting is a very human skill. So, a piece of meat that has been fried or a baked potato are both 'processed', in that they are no longer raw. They have been through a process – in this case, of being heated up and cooked. Likewise, a can of peaches, a jar of chutney, a piece of smoked fish, or a wedge of Brie are all examples of foods that have been processed. But none of them is 'ultra-processed'. Ultra-processing is a much more modern technique, in which raw ingredients are worked on in a factory setting to the point that they often become unrecognizable, with other ingredients – not derived from food at all – then added in order to maximize profit.

The term 'ultra-processed food' was coined by Brazilian nutritionist Carlos Monteiro in 2009[2] and, along with a team of researchers, he then developed the four-part Nova classification to try to bring more clarity to nutrition and public health.[3] It's worth remembering that Monteiro's categories were never developed for shoppers and consumers looking to decide whether or not to eat individual items. They were created to help researchers categorize foods in groups in order to assess their impact on our diets. Some think they are therefore a bit of a blunt instrument and can make people anxious about their choices. My personal view is that they are a good place to start (and then nuance needs to be introduced, and we'll come to that on page 25). So here goes:

SO, WHAT IS ULTRA-PROCESSED FOOD (UPF)?

The four Nova categories are:

Nova 1: Unprocessed or minimally processed foods
The foods in this category have had nothing or next-to-nothing done to change them. Examples of minimal processing include chopping, freezing, drying or packaging. This means they are unlikely to have an ingredients label. These are single-ingredient items. Examples: eggs, raw meat, vegetables, fruit, nuts, milk, spices, canned fruit or veg with nothing added.

Nova 2: Processed culinary ingredients (sometimes called 'oils, fats, salts and sugar')
The foods in his category have been extracted from Nova 1 foods or from nature. They are not normally consumed by themselves. They will probably have a label, but may not state ingredients – and if ingredients are stated, they should still only have one. Examples: butter, salt, sugar, honey, olive oil, maple syrup.

Nova 3: Processed foods
The foods in this category have been made by combining foods from Nova 1 and Nova 2 and putting them through processes like baking, fermenting, boiling or canning. But they should have only two or three ingredients. Examples: tinned tuna (tuna, olive oil); Cheddar cheese (milk); home-made biscuits (flour, sugar, butter); bakery/artisan/homemade bread (flour, water, yeast, salt, olive oil); cured meat; pickled vegetables.

Nova 4: Ultra-processed foods

The foods in this category usually have a high number of ingredients, including some not used in home cooking, such as emulsifiers, stabilisers and antioxidants, and usually with no intact foods from Nova 1. They are 'industrial formulations', made using substances derived from food combined with a huge variety of additives. Examples: fizzy drinks, ice cream, bread and cakes (industrially made), ready meals, plant-based 'meat' and 'milk', crisps.

Nova Group 1	**Unprocessed or minimally processed foods:** edible parts of plants (e.g. apples) or animals (e.g. lamb chop), with very little done to change them.
Nova Group 2	**Processed culinary ingredients (oils, fats, salts and sugar):** derived from Nova Group 1 foods or from nature, minimally processed so that you can prepare other dishes with them, e.g. flour, butter, sugar, oils.
Nova Group 3	**Processed foods:** usually made from combining Nova Group 1 and Nova Group 2, e.g. cheese, pickles, artisan bread.
Nova Group 4	**Ultra-processed foods (UPFs):** Factory-made food-like products that bear little resemblance to Nova Group 1 foods, e.g. cola, cake bars, ready meals.

SO, WHAT IS ULTRA-PROCESSED FOOD (UPF)?

How will you recognize Nova Group 4 foods when you are shopping? Here's some examples of labels to help give you a sense of what you're looking for. I've put the ingredients in bold that I would consider to be indicative of UPF – I definitely don't have any of them in my kitchen!

Batchelors BBQ Beef Super Noodles

Noodles (80%) (Wheat Flour, **Palm Oil, Potato Starch, Acidity Regulators (Potassium Lactate, Citric Acid)**, Salt, **Flavour Enhancer (Monosodium Glutamate), Colour (Carotenes), Antioxidant (Tocopherol-Rich Extract), Stabiliser (Potassium Carbonate), Flour Treatment Agent (Sodium Carbonate)), Maltodextrin,** Wheat Flour, **Maize Starch, Flavourings (contain Milk),** Dried Peas (1%), **Yeast Extract,** Dried Carrot (0.5%), **Flavour Enhancers (Monosodium Glutamate, Disodium 5'-Ribonucleotides),** Onion Powder, **Milk Mineral Concentrate,** Salt, **Colours (Plain Caramel, Paprika Extract), Thickener (Guar Gum),** Thyme Extract, **Acid (Citric Acid), Black Pepper Extract,** Sugar, Parsley, **Smoke Flavourings.**

Tesco Wholemeal Bread

Wholemeal Wheat Flour, Water, Yeast, Salt, Barley Malt Flour, Sugar, **Emulsifiers (Mono- and Diacetyl Tartaric Acid Esters of Mono- and Diglycerides of Fatty Acids, Mono- and Diglycerides of Fatty Acids),** Spirit Vinegar, **Preservative (Calcium Propionate),** Rapeseed Oil, **Wheat Gluten, Flour Treatment Agent (Ascorbic Acid).**

Sour Cream and Onion Pringles

Dehydrated Potatoes, Vegetable Oils (Sunflower, **Palm**, Corn) in varying proportions, Wheat Flour, Corn Flour, Rice Flour, **Sour Cream & Onion Seasoning** (Onion Powder, Wheat Starch, Maltodextrin, Flavour Enhancers {Monosodium Glutamate, Disodium Guanylate, Disodium Inosinate}, Dextrose, Sunflower Oil, Salt, Flavourings {Milk}, Sugar, Sour Cream Powder {Milk}, Modified Maize Starch, Sweet Whey Powder {Milk}, Glucose Syrup, Acids {Citric Acid, Lactic Acid, Malic Acid}, Milk Proteins), Maltodextrin, Emulsifier (E471), Salt, Colour (**Annatto Norbixin**).

Go Ahead Fruit & Oat Bakes

Apple Flavoured Filling (43%) [Glucose Syrup, Humectant (Glycerine), Glucose-Fructose Syrup, Apple Juice Concentrate (1.8%), Wheat Dextrin, Acidity Regulators (Citric Acid, Malic Acid, Calcium Citrates), Gelling Agents (Pectins, Sodium Alginate), Vegetable Fibre, Thickener (Modified Starch), Natural Apple Flavouring], Flour (Wheat Flour, Calcium, Iron, Niacin, Thiamin), Oatmeal (11%), Sugar, Vegetable Oil (Sunflower), Water, **Maltodextrin, Partially Inverted Sugar Syrup, Polydextrose,** Starch, Invert Sugar Syrup, Wheat Gluten, Salt, Raising Agents (Sodium Bicarbonate, **Disodium Diphosphate**), Emulsifiers (Soya Lecithin, E472e), Natural Flavouring.

SO, WHAT IS ULTRA-PROCESSED FOOD (UPF)?

Ambrosia Plant Based Custard

Water, Sugar, **Modified Starch, Sustainable Palm Oil, Inulin, Emulsifiers (Sucrose Esters of Fatty Acids, Lecithin), Calcium Phosphate,** Salt, **Stabilisers (Xanthan Gum, Carrageenan), Natural Flavourings, Colours (Carotenes, Paprika Extract).**

Waitrose Essentials Coconut Milk

Coconut extract (60%), Water, **Stabilisers (guar gum and carboxy methyl cellulose), Emulsifier (sucrose esters of fatty acids).**

Philadelphia Cream Cheese

Full Fat Soft Cheese, Salt, **Stabiliser (Guar Gum), Acid (Citric Acid).**

Activia Gut Health Low Fat Yogurt and Granola

Vanilla Yogurt (88%): Yogurt (Milk), Water, Sugar (5, 5%), **Natural Flavouring,** Vanilla, **Acidity Regulators (Citric Acid, Calcium Citrate), Modified Starch, Stabilisers (Pectin, Guar Gum), Colouring (Beta Carotene, Curcumin),** Cereal Clusters (12%): Oat Flakes, Sugar, Cereal Crispies (Maize, Rice, Sugar, Whole Wheat Flour, Rye, Barley, Barley Malt, Low Fat Cocoa Powder, Salt), Sunflower Oil, Wheat Flour, Rye Flour, Wheat Germ, Coconut Flakes, **Dextrose,** Honey, Salt.

Oh, so you don't just mean junk food then?

Unfortunately, no, not really – that would be simple! In fact, there's a common misconception that if it's expensive or upmarket in any way, it's not UPF. This really isn't the case – there are plenty of higher-end items that tick the UPF box: fancy cakes, luxury lunch salads, posh crisps, top-of-the-range ready meals, to name a few examples. And whilst it's probably safe to say that all junk food is ultra-processed, it doesn't therefore follow that all UPFs are what we perceive as junk food. For example, not many of us think of a loaf of sliced bread as junk food, and yet almost all factory-made, supermarket bread – a staple of many of our diets – is ultra-processed. Likewise, breakfast cereals, which many of us have grown up being told are a 'healthy start' to the day, are almost all UPF, and so are most of the 'healthy' yoghurts, and so are cereal snack bars.

To complicate things further, many foods that are classified as Nova category 3, or 'processed', when made at home or on a small scale, are considered Nova 4 – and therefore UPFs – when produced industrially. Examples include bread, pizza, biscuits, and cake. The scale of UPF production is mind-boggling – on a single day in the UK alone, over 3,000 factories churn out 12 million loaves of bread and 10 million cakes and biscuits.[4] The methods we might use to make a cake at home with butter, sugar, flour and eggs just don't translate to mass production. So the butter and sugar are replaced with much cheaper fats and sweeteners, and emulsifiers, flavourings and preservatives are added to give it a convincing taste and texture, and often a mind-bogglingly distant 'use by' date. If you've ever made bread at home or bought an 'artisan' loaf, you'll know it's the same story – they go stale much more quickly. So, in go the UPF ingredients for regularity of taste and texture and maximum shelf-life and profit. In fact, UPF products have become so widespread that it's much harder to find a product that is *not* UPF – they are floor-to-ceiling in almost every aisle.

Confused?

Perhaps it would help if we took a quick tour round the nearest supermarket? **But first, a word about nuance...**

To make things clear, especially for people who are new to the idea of UPF, it's easiest to start with a black-and-white approach: yes this item *is* UPF, no this item is *not*. But as you progress through your own journey of thinking differently about food, you may find that there are some grey areas where you feel the health benefits or even the convenience of a particular item outweighs the concern that it may be UPF. Perhaps it just has one ingredient you don't recognize. Maybe your child is a fussy eater and you know this is something they won't object to. Or maybe it's something like a stock cube and you're going to add it to a fantastic home-cooked meal. And, as I said in the Introduction, it's not just about reading the ingredients list and saying yay or nay – we need to reconsider our relationship with what we eat and reintroduce values of gratitude and mindfulness to our diet. But we have to understand what UPF is first, and then we can introduce some nuance and decide what approach we are going to take. It's a journey. There are more thoughts about this in Chapter

12 (see page 253), but for now…let's grab a trolley and through the supermarket doors we go.

FRUIT & VEG

In almost every such shop around the world, the first things you will encounter are the fresh stuff, like fruit, veg, meat, cheese and milk. We're not going to get sidetracked by discussions over organic, free-range, etc. – on this trip round the shop we're only going to think about one question: what is UPF? So for now, you can safely put as many heads of broccoli or bags of apples in your trolley as you like, they are minimally processed (trimmed, chopped and packaged), but they are not UPF.

MEAT & FISH

Likewise in this aisle, you can put your chicken fillets or tuna steaks into the trolley without a UPF-related care in the world: again, it has been minimally processed – if it hadn't, it would still be mooing at you or covered in feathers. Watch out, though, for meat that has been coated or marinated, for example boxes of ribs or wings, because if you check the ingredients, you're likely to find preservatives, thickeners and syrups that take you into UPF territory.

DAIRY

As we round the bend into the dairy aisle, things start to get even more complicated. Cow's milk, fine. Traditional cheese, fine. But if you like to buy your cheese ready grated, it's not 'just cheese', it's got extras like anti-caking agents and potato starch added, to stop it sticking together in the pack. Cream cheese might be okay, but some brands contain stabilisers like 'guar gum', 'carrageenan' and even 'citrus fibre', and likewise those cheese triangles you stick in the kids' lunch boxes have extras like 'phosphates' and 'inulin'.

You might regularly add yoghurt to your trolley, but unless it's unflavoured, natural yoghurt, I have bad news – it's UPF, because it's thickened with modified maize starch, sweetened with sugar or artificial sweeteners and made 'creamier', not with cream, but with gums, oils and powders.

CHILLED FOODS

As we venture further into the chilled section, things take a turn for the worse: as you might expect, the ready meals, sausage rolls, quiches and pizzas, and quite a lot of the sausages and 'reformed' meats, all contain ingredients you would not find in your home kitchen, from bamboo fibre to palm oil to antioxidants, all added to increase shelf-life. Salted, dried and cured meat and fish don't count as UPF – although you may wish to check the ingredients for any rogue additives or flavourings.

BAKERY

Bad news, too, in the bakery aisle – cakes and biscuits were probably the pioneers of UPF, with 'shop-bought' pancake mixes being marketed as early as the turn of the twentieth century, and brands like Betty Crocker and Mr Kipling becoming household names in the post-war era. If you've ever made cakes or biscuits at home, you'll know they are all iterations of four basic components: flour, sugar, butter and eggs. But check the ingredients of the Mini Rolls, Oreos and Twinkies and you'll find a whole host of extras that you do not have in your baking cupboard: palm and rapeseed oil, glucose-fructose syrup, soya lecithin, gums and emulsifiers.

Bread, too, is almost all UPF. In fact, 'bread' is a somewhat disputed word in itself, as are the terms 'fresh', 'freshly baked' and 'sourdough'. The Real Bread Campaign in the UK says there are barely any restrictions on what can be labelled as bread. They told me: 'The Bread and Flour Regulations state: bread means a food of any size, shape or form which simply has to be, "usually known as bread" and "consist of a dough made from flour and water, with or without other ingredients, which has been fermented by yeast or otherwise leavened and subsequently baked or partly baked".'

They also noted that 'There are no legal definitions, and no regulation, of commonly used marketing terms including: wholegrain, sourdough, artisan, or heritage wheat.' (Not so in France, where the Décret Pain (Bread Decree) of 1993 stated that traditional baguettes must be made on the premises where they are sold and can only be made with four ingredients: wheat flour, water, salt and yeast, with no additives or preservatives.) If you've ever made bread yourself, you'll know it's basically just as the French have decreed: flour, yeast, water and salt. And you'll know that, like a true French stick, it only keeps for a day or two before drying out. But your sliced supermarket loaf is something different – a fluffy concoction of all kinds of other ingredients, including the inevitable palm and rapeseed oils, soya flour, and something known as DATEM (Diacetyl tartaric acid ester of mono- and diglycerides, also E472e), which gives each slice that springy, moreish texture, even when it's been sat in your bread bin for a week or so.

Other products that take a mysteriously long time to go off, like pre-packed wraps, crumpets, bagels and brioche, all contain extra ingredients that you would definitely not be adding were you to bake them at home. Let's take brioche as an example. Make it in your own kitchen and you'll need: flour, sugar, yeast, eggs, milk, butter and a pinch of salt. Buy it in the supermarket and it will contain all these things, plus a few extras like: rapeseed oil, mono- and diglycerides of fatty acids, hydrolysed wheat protein, a thickener called caroboxymethylcellulose, flavouring, milk proteins, a colour called beta-carotene and the antioxidant ascorbic acid. (These ingredients are listed on Tesco brioche butter rolls.)

SNACKS

Push that trolley round the corner into the snack section and you probably won't be surprised to learn that UPF abounds. Crisps – well, many of them are not even made from sliced potatoes, but instead are made of what the manufacturers optimistically call 'dough', which is a mushy mix of starches, oils and emulsifiers, reformed into different shapes depending on the brand, baked or fried, and then coated in another mix of flavourings, sugars and preservatives. The only ones that don't seem to fall into the UPF category are some (but not all) brands of 'ready salted', with just potato, oil and salt. Although the ready salted of the leading UK brand, Walkers, also contains four different antioxidants to prevent the crisps going rancid. Other snacks such as flavoured nuts and popcorn are UPF, and don't let's even go there with 'cereal bars', which often make bold health or diet claims on the packaging but are usually packed with sugar syrups, palm and other oils, emulsifiers, and gums.

Most chocolate bars, too, are UPF, and they are not immune from health claims, either. Cadbury's Dairy Milk marketed itself for decades with the image of a 'glass & a half of milk in every bar', but read the small print and you'll find that this translates to 426ml of milk in every 227g of chocolate. Look closer: 426ml is about two highball glasses; 227g is the weight of more than four individual bars. So that's less than 100ml of milk per bar – about half a champagne flute. I'm not sure which type of glass Cadbury's was working from. In 2010, EU regulations meant Cadbury's had to stop using the words 'glass & a half of milk' on its wrappers,[5] but interestingly it was allowed to keep the image, and a few years later it launched an ad campaign about the 'Glass and a Half in Everyone', ostensibly about the goodness in people but presumably also an excellent way to reinforce the idea of wholesome milky

SO, WHAT IS ULTRA-PROCESSED FOOD (UPF)?

chocolate. As well as milk, a Dairy Milk bar contains a few less wholesome ingredients: palm oil and shea oil plus two different E numbers: the emulsifier E442, which keeps the cocoa butter and powder from separating, and E476, which improves something called 'mouth feel'; in other words, you can put less of the expensive cocoa butter in and still get that nice melty, creamy texture.

DRY INGREDIENTS & CONDIMENTS

Anyway, put that chocolate back on the shelf and let's push our trolley round to the store-cupboard aisle with the dry ingredients, jars of sauce, condiments and tins. Here we find a mixed bag: pasta, rice, and couscous are all processed but *not* UPF – because they don't contain any 'hidden extras' – whereas noodles need a bit more scrutiny, particularly any that come with sachets of flavouring. Pulses and vegetables in tins are usually 'just what it says on the tin', although it's worth reading the label. Tinned soups, however, are almost all UPF, containing the usual suspects like modified maize starch, maltodextrin, sugars, oils and gums, depending on the brand. Baked beans and ketchup, those staples of the British diet, are both surprisingly free of these extra ingredients, but not so my favourite condiment, mayonnaise in a jar, many brands of which contain a preservative called EDTA. This is a chemical additive that's a 'chelating agent' – meaning it binds to metals and prevents them from becoming part of any chemical reactions. This metal-binding ability means that EDTA is also used in face cream (see page 216) and injected to treat lead and mercury poisoning, which I don't know about you but has put me right off my club sandwich.

BREAKFAST CEREALS

Moving on to the breakfast cereal section – as previously mentioned, this is a hotbed of UPF, and the very fact that we've been convinced into eating it every morning for one of our three meals of the day is a testament to twentieth-century food marketers. The only ones you are safe to put in your fictional trolley are porridge oats, Shredded Wheat, Weetabix, some mueslis and, if you must, Corn Flakes and Bran Flakes, which at least don't contain the bulking agents, palm oils, syrups, emulsifiers and antioxidants of most of cereals on offer on these shelves. The ones that kids are attracted to are usually the worst – if it's got a bug-eyed cartoon character on the front and it claims it's 'great for brain development' or 'packed with added goodness', then avoid it like the plague.

FROZEN FOODS

As you might expect, the convenience foods that the freezer section is packed with are mostly UPF, with pizzas and ready meals being the most obvious suspects. But even 'healthy'-sounding products like 'Honey Roast Parsnips' can contain rapeseed, sunflower and palm oil, rice flour, maize flour, dextrin, raising agents (diphosphates and sodium carbonate) and xanthan gum. Ice cream – which if you've made it at home you will know is pretty much 'iced cream' (cream, sugar, vanilla, sometimes eggs) – is a UPF disaster zone, packed with emulsifiers, thickeners, sweeteners, oils and gums.

THE BOOZE

Shall we put some drinks in our trolley before we check out? Don't worry, I'm not going to ruin your day by telling you that wine is a UPF. If we're just using the Nova categories to decide (and I felt this to be so important that I checked with Carlos Monteiro, who originated Nova), then both wine and beer would technically be a Nova 3, or 'processed', because they still bear a resemblance to the original foods they are derived from, for example grapes in the case of wine and grains in the case of beer. But according to Monteiro and Nova, spirits like whisky, gin and vodka would be Nova 4, or 'ultra processed', because they are so far from the original food they are made from. Where wine and beer are only fermented, spirits are then distilled, and this extra process makes them UPF.

In my opinion, this all bears a bit more scrutiny and nuance. Living in Somerset as I do, just down the road from a cider farm, I can tell you there is a world of difference between the drink they make from fermented apples and the popular brands of commercially produced fizzy cider made by adding fermented corn starch syrup to cheap apple juice along with a host of additives. Likewise, real ale is very different in make-up from mass-produced lager, and when it comes to wine there are also options like organic and sulphite-free. You need to use your own discernment and decide what is important to you and how much you are going to be drinking (bearing in mind that alcohol in excess is not great for health).

When it comes to spirits, it seems hard to believe that an artisan Scotch whisky, made to the same recipe for hundreds of years, is in the same category as a pot noodle. Again, this is a matter for your own judgement, but if it's additives and preservatives you are most concerned about, you're better off avoiding flavoured spirits, canned cocktails and alcopops. And if you want a soft drink, your best bet is to stick to water. Almost all fizzy drinks, squashes, energy drinks and flavoured waters could be described as ultra-processed, including those that are 'diet' and those with 'zero' calories or other health claims. Of all the items we have debated over putting in our trolley, there is barely any argument that can be made for their inclusion in our diet – we just don't need them. There'll be plenty more mentions of fizzy drinks later in the book, but for now, let's head for the checkouts...

Err...wait a second...my trolley is looking pretty empty, and I've left a lot of my favourite snacks on the shelves. What exactly is the problem with UPF?

The problem seems to be, put simply, that *we were never meant to eat this stuff.* It may be 'edible', but, when you think about it, so is craft glue, face cream, paper, chalk and crayons (in small quantities, but don't try this at home, folks!). You could even eat a house brick if you felt inclined. But being able to put something in your mouth, chew it, swallow it and survive is not really what defines something as 'food'. It has to be nutritious, but it also has to *not* be the opposite – i.e.

detrimental to our health. And there is growing evidence that UPFs, which humans have only been consuming for around fifty years (not long when you consider we've been on the planet for millennia), and which are becoming more and more ubiquitous in our diets, are causing us real harm.

2.

What's the problem with UPF?

And why are we suddenly talking about it now?

If you're feeling a bit blindsided by suddenly being asked to overhaul the entire way you shop, cook and eat, it might help to know that the idea that UPF is bad for us isn't as new as all that. In fact, as things so often do, it's happened slowly and then all at once. It might surprise you to discover that our current conversation about UPF has not only already been had, but that it also contains repeating patterns that usually involve anyone raising concerns being thoroughly discredited. In the Western world at least, humans began to industrially process food as long ago as the 1940s in response to the crisis of the Second World War and the subsequent hardship that followed. And even then, concerns were raised about the impact on health of what was then called 'highly processed food'. For example, Dr Noah Philip Norman and his co-author James Rorty declared it a 'fad' and 'not really food at all' in their 1947 book *Tomorrow's Food*. They called for a consumer boycott, but were labelled 'pseudoscientists', and the food-processing conveyor-belt whirred onwards. In the early 1950s the advent of the TV dinner offered the idea that UPF could liberate women from the drudgery of the kitchen, and by the early 1970s so-called 'junk food' was a familiar part of the Western diet.

Again and again, doctors, writers and activists raised the alarm and were discredited, often by those on the payroll of the food industry itself. Further resistance came in the form of ideas about 'holistic medicine', chiming with other concerns in the zeitgeist over nuclear war and the environment. In 1975 a 'Food Day' was organized, with events across the USA, to put forward the argument that minimally processed foods should be accessible and available to all. One of the organizers, nutrition professor Dr Joan Dye Gussow, told a crowd that highly processed food was not really food at all and called for a return to whole, minimally processed food: 'No one has taken it and boiled it and smashed it and fortified it and extruded it and baked it and sugared it and dyed it lilac and put it into a four-coloured printed box and called it Wonder Bear, or Mr. Whammy, or Purple Elephant Flakes, or Instant Anything. And we are better off because they haven't. It is time we all got back to eating food again.'

Fifty years later, the story of Food Day seems to keep repeating itself: grassroots protest against the damage of UPF, followed by backlash and discreditation from the food industries. Food Day was slammed for 'creating anxiety by disseminating misinformation' and condemned as 'hairbrained' – but the leading voices of condemnation were all on the payroll of multinational brands who stood to lose billions if the likes of Joan Gussow were taken seriously.

So why are we all talking about UPF again now?

In the 1970s it might have been easy to dismiss food activists as hippies and killjoys, but now something new has happened that we simply have to take note of: many countries of the world have seen a huge uptick in both obesity and non-communicable diseases such as cancer, heart disease and diabetes. Climate change has also forced us to think about the 'bigger picture' and to ask more questions about how our food is produced and what its impact might be, not just on our own bodies but on the future of the planet. Added to this, the work of two different experts, Carlos Monteiro in Brazil and Kevin Hall in the USA, has shifted the conversation about UPF forwards in ways that are no longer so easy to ignore.

In 2009, motivated by the rising rates of obesity and Type 2 diabetes in Brazil, Carlos Monteiro and his team proposed the four Nova groups we saw in Chapter 1 (see table, page 20), which created a whole new way of classifying food based on how much it has been processed and why. This cemented the term 'ultra-processed foods' in our lexicon, although it had been used before. In the 1980s, for example, the writer Laurence Shames (now best known for his comic mystery novels) wrote a piece in *Esquire* on unethical marketing and described 'ultra-processed foodstuffs whose labels read like a chem text'. But Monteiro's work doesn't just name or criticize UPF, it clearly defines what it is, and this is key: you cannot effectively research what you cannot classify. Monteiro's work led to many observational studies, but not everyone was initially convinced that UPF was the culprit for global health problems, with some questioning whether it's simply the high levels of fat and sugar in UPF that we should be addressing, rather than the processing itself. What was needed was the gold standard in evidence: a randomized controlled trial.

Step forward nutrition researcher Kevin Hall, who in 2016 first heard the idea that UPF was responsible for obesity and thought it was a load of pre-packed baloney. He believed people like Monteiro were getting it wrong, and that it was probably the economic brackets and lifestyles of people who were most likely to be eating large amounts of UPF that were driving weight gain, rather than UPF itself. He wanted to prove that it wasn't the processing of food that mattered, but only the nutritional content – fat, sugar, salt and fibre – and that a person eating the right balance of these would be just fine, whether the stuff they were eating was ultra-processed or not. In 2019 he set up a trial to test this, recruiting ten men and ten women to spend four weeks living in a clinic and eating a diet prescribed by Hall and his team.[1] For two weeks, half the group ate a diet consisting entirely of UPF, whilst the other half ate unprocessed meals cooked from scratch – and then they swapped. Hall and his team worked hard to ensure that the nutritional content of their meals was as equivalent as possible in terms of fat, sugar, salt and fibre, and participants were allowed to eat as much or as little of each type of diet as they chose. The results were seismic, forcing Hall to rethink his scepticism, and signifying a global turning-point in attitudes, too. On the UPF diet, participants:

- ate around 500 more calories per day;
- gained around 2 lbs (or 1 kg) over the two weeks on the diet;
- ate their food more quickly;
- had lower levels of the appetite-suppressing hormone (PYY) and higher levels of the hunger hormone (ghrelin) than when eating the unprocessed diet.

Hall's research results suggested that Monteiro might have been right about the link between UPF and obesity – when eating UPF, even though participants could choose how much they ate, they ate faster, ate more, and gained weight. The trial also suggested that there was something very different about the way this type of food interacts with the human body. Whilst it might be nutritionally identical, with the same protein, fat, sugar and calories, the body seems to be doing one thing when we eat an ultra-processed pizza, and something else when we eat a homemade pizza. This upends decades of thinking about 'bad food', 'good food' and 'healthy eating' – because it tells us that it's not specific dishes or foods that we should avoid or be cautious of, but the way they are created.

Why we eat more of this type of food than we need is a question that experts are still exploring – although if you've ever sat down in front of the telly with a tube of Pringles and found you've rapidly demolished the lot, you may already intuitively know the answer. UPFs are hyperpalatable. They taste great, they are loaded with salts and sugars that get our palates excited, they have enticing packaging, they have enjoyable textures, and they make us crave another, then another, then another. As the Pringles slogan literally tells us in a rare moment of honesty: *Once you pop, you can't stop!* When my kids ask for a snack and I say, 'If you're hungry, have an apple', they groan and roll their eyes – because they're not hungry for an apple. Apples are hard work compared to a salty, umami packet of cheese puffs that melt on your tongue, or a soft and enticing pre-packed mini cake that delivers that quick and easy sugar hit. Our kids know it, and we know it too.

What does the evidence say?

The groundbreaking work of Monteiro and Hall paved the way for a multitude of studies. A global team of researchers recently conducted the world's largest ever review of the evidence around UPF, looking at everything published over the past three years and involving almost ten million participants. This research was not funded by any company involved in the production of UPF. Its findings were published in the *British Medical Journal* in February 2024.[2] Researchers found links between UPF and 32 harmful effects to health, including a higher risk of heart disease, cancer, Type 2 diabetes, adverse mental health and early death.

They found 'convincing evidence' of an association between a higher exposure to UPF and:
- 50 per cent increased risk of cardiovascular disease-related death;
- 48–53 per cent higher risk of anxiety and common mental disorders;

- 12 per cent greater risk of Type 2 diabetes.

They found 'highly suggestive' evidence of a link between higher UPF consumption and:
- 21 per cent greater risk of death from any cause;
- 40–66 per cent increased risk of heart disease-related death, obesity, Type 2 diabetes, and sleep problems;
- 22 per cent increased risk of depression.

And when it comes to the female body, other studies have found links between UPF and:
- more painful and heavier periods,[3] and worse symptoms of PMS;[4]
- increased symptoms of menopause;[5]
- 50 per cent higher risk of depression in middle-age women;[6]
- increased risk of developing and dying from female cancers;[7]
- higher risk of health problems in pregnancy;[8]
- increased risk of dementia and Alzheimer's.[9]

Is there still a push back against the idea that UPF is to blame?

Yes. Monteiro's Nova scale, for example, has been criticized, with some suggesting it's too complicated for people to categorize their food in this way. Others say that people will just not have the time or the money to cook with fresh raw ingredients – and that life without UPF is simply impossible.

But it is worth remembering that every time we see resistance to the idea that UPF might be driving a public health crisis, there are huge multinational companies who stand to lose if we change our eating habits. Some compare the current situation with UPF to the way tobacco companies worked hard for decades to downplay the risks of smoking – and in fact there are literal overlaps: food giant Kraft was owned by tobacco giant Philip Morris until 2007. Although our supermarkets may seem to be filled with a huge variety of brands, in reality almost all of them come under the umbrella of just ten huge global corporations: Nestlé, PepsiCo, Coca-Cola, Unilever, Danone, Kellogg's, Ferrero, Mars, KraftHeinz and Mondelēz, International. If you read a news article or even a piece of research that questions whether UPF is something we should be concerned about, it's worth asking if there were any of these big food brands involved in the background. Likewise, if you pick up a UPF product in a shop, it's worth asking: who will gain if I eat this product? And what was the main motivation of the company who will receive money when I buy it?

Why is food being made like this?

The short answer is: profit. Going back to that apple that our time-traveller would recognize in the grocery store but that my kids are not really craving when they want a snack – it may be delicious and healthy, but it's difficult to make money out of it. But if you take that apple and make it into concentrated fruit purée, you can then add it into a whole range of other products, whilst leaning heavily on the inherent 'healthy' associations we all have with apples and fruit in general. The packaging of the Go Ahead Fruit & Oat Bakes that my kids would much prefer at snack time, for example, tells me that they are 'Golden Baked Oaty Bars with an Apple Flavoured Filling'. Glance at the back of the pack and it says the 'apple filling' is 43 per cent of the ingredients. But dig a bit deeper and you'll find that this most certainly doesn't mean that the bars are 43 per cent apple. In fact, that 'filling' is mainly made with a rogues' gallery of UPF ingredients: glucose syrup, glycerine, wheat dextrin, three different 'acidity regulators', two different 'gelling agents', vegetable fibre, thickener, apple flavouring and, oh, 1.8 per cent of it is 'apple juice concentrate'. And that's just the filling. The rest of the bar, the 'oaty' bit, is only 11 per cent oatmeal – and bear in mind that 'oatmeal' is what you get when you process oats into a sort of flour. And then the UPF ingredients just keep stacking up: sugar, maltodextrin, partially inverted sugar syrup, polydextrose, starch, invert sugar syrup, wheat gluten, salt, two different raising agents, and two emulsifiers (soya lecithin, and E472e – otherwise known as DATEM – see page 29). The bars contain over 30 different ingredients – most of them a million miles away from the 'fruit and oat' they are named after – that give them an extra-long shelf-life and a good profit margin. In spite of the label, you are not really eating much 'fruit' or 'oats' at all, and any apple you are eating is highly processed, which means it is not having the same effect on your body as, say, a slice of real apple, because its molecular structure is completely different. This is what scientists call the 'food matrix'.

When it comes to the crunch

OK, what's the food matrix? Surely apples are apples are apples? Not quite. The molecular structure of food changes depending on what we do to it, and it's this structure that is referred to as its 'matrix'. So, a raw, hard, crunchy apple will have a different matrix or molecular structure from apple sauce, and apple sauce a different matrix from a golden baked oaty bar with apple flavoured filling. We change the matrix of our food when we grind it, mix it and cook it, and have been doing so for millennia. But only recently have scientists begun to explore how foods that are literally 'the same' in terms of ingredients and nutritional content, for example nuts and ground nuts, can not only have a different matrix but can impact the body in different ways, depending on their matrix. Whole almonds, for example, have a structure made of fibrous cell walls with fat globules inside. When you eat them, the fat stays within the cell walls and is not absorbed by the body. Grind up the same quantity of almonds and you get a different matrix because the cell walls are broken and the fat released – meaning they deliver around 30 per cent more calories to the body than whole nuts, and cause the levels of fat in your blood to rise more rapidly.

The matrix is the reason why scientists are now beginning to warn that fruit juices may not, in fact, be 'healthy', in particular if we consume a lot of them, because the juicing breaks down the cell walls in the fruit, removing its fibre and allowing its sugars to be absorbed much more rapidly by the body. This can cause an unhealthy spike in your blood sugar, followed by a sudden drop, and if these spikes and drops are repeated over time, they can damage your metabolic health and increase your chances of Type 2 diabetes and obesity. Put simply, you are far better off eating a whole piece of fruit. Obviously, the more a food is processed, the more the food matrix is disrupted and changed, so with UPF, where the original apple or nut is almost impossible to recognize, we are only just beginning to understand how the body responds.

It's also true that when my kids eat their 'oat bar' or 'Fruit Winder', it's not just about what they are eating – it's also about what they are *not* eating: that apple, with its particularly crunchy matrix, sits abandoned in the fruit bowl. UPF may fill us up, but it's also depriving us of something – all of that whole food that we are not eating. The science is complex and emerging on this, but what we can safely say is that we are some of the first humans on the planet to eat stuff with this particular UPF matrix, and the first to eat a lot *fewer* whole foods with their particular and very different matrix. It's a bit of an experiment and, so far, the results don't seem to be great.

So, we have a problem – what now?

When I first started really delving into the topic of UPF, I felt completely overwhelmed. I can still remember one evening supermarket dash, knowing that everyone would be arriving home soon and that the fridge was empty. 'I don't have time to make some organic bloody lentil flipping atrocity that my kids won't eat,' I muttered darkly to myself as I pushed my trolley around the aisles. Two experiences I already found stressful – the overstimulating, brightly lit supermarket, and thinking up 'meal plans' for our family of two adults and three children, one of whom has severe allergies – now had a whole new layer to add: UPF. When I'd first read about UPF, I hadn't been particularly worried. We cook a lot in our house, and I'd assumed we were already consuming a fairly low amount of it. But then I started reading labels – something I was already well-versed in with a child with allergies in the house – looking at every packet and tin and asking new questions: do I have these ingredients in my kitchen? Is that just a fancy word for salt or is it made in some industrial vat somewhere? WTF is carrageenan? My eyes began to ache from it all.

I wandered the aisles that night, ostensibly searching for a quick family dinner but presumably looking somewhat deranged. It was as if a really horrible UPF lightbulb had been switched on, illuminating a whole load of things I'd rather not see. What was once just a bog-standard stressful experience had taken on a kind of existential malaise. 'What on Earth are we all doing here?', I wanted to shout to the all the other zombie shoppers. 'Wake up!!' All of the plastic packaging, the chemical additives, the bread that isn't really bread, the puddings in trays, the fridge raiders, the palm oil in *everything*, the crisps that aren't potato…even the tins of chickpeas I thought made me some kind of home cookery master contained an 'antioxidant' called 'ascorbic acid'. 'DOES THIS MAKE THEM UPF?', I wanted to yell at the hideous ceiling lights. I already had what felt like an unreasonable number of worries – now I had to add saving the bloody planet and my family's health by soaking pulses overnight and making my own flipping hummus. I left that night with a stack of frozen pizzas, a cheap bottle of pinot grigio, and a feeling of defeat.

Whether or not you share my sense of overwhelm, I think we can all agree that any conversation about UPF has absolutely got to acknowledge the woman this scenario represents: her valuable time, her mental health, her bandwidth for learning, her capacity for change, her budget. UPF cannot be yet another man-made problem that women are expected to fix, adding the weight of finding solutions – and the inevitable guilt and shame of frequently being unable to – to our already heavy load. If we are going to 'get back in the kitchen', then we need to do so in ways that work for us, and make sure that the men in our lives are there alongside us this time, pulling their weight. The vast majority of celebrity chefs are male, and over 75 per cent of professional chefs are male. Quitting or reducing UPF is going to mean men bringing some of those talents into the home kitchen. As well as this, corporations need to step up. At the time of writing, the CEO of every major global food company in the world is a man. These companies need to listen to women and offer us solutions for the family table that are time-saving without being toxic.

The price of resistance

And what about cost? We mentioned budget above and this is another argument made against change – food companies would probably very much like us to believe the story that a non-UPF diet will cost us more. This was actually reinforced by Kevin Hall's research (remember the groups that ate UPF and non-UPF for four weeks and the UPF eaters ate 500 calories more and put on weight? See page 40). Hall's researchers spent 40 per cent more preparing the non-UPF diet, a fact that is oft-repeated – but they were dishing up meals like prime cuts of meat and fish.

If you want to replicate your pre-UPF life, which probably involved a wide variety of cuisines and choices, plenty of meat, cakes and biscuits on demand, and complex hot meals ready in minutes, then this will not only be difficult but also costly. But it's also these high expectations that many of us have grown up with, of having so many different recipes made for us, and being convinced that they are just as nutritious as if we had made them ourselves, that are the costly part of UPF. The frozen pizzas I bought after my existential crisis probably cost more per head than a pizza made from scratch, but I, and now my kids as well, have been sold all kinds of ideas about those pizzas (they are a treat, they are delicious, they are balanced, they are from a 'Ristorante', they are Italian), most of which probably isn't true. In fact, they tasted pretty revolting after the first couple of mouthfuls. If I'd wanted to be truly Mediterranean, I could probably have bought some pasta and served it with olive oil, cheese, ham and a few bits of salad for the same price and level of cooking effort. But the pizza looked good on the packaging and the branding implied it was fresh out of Naples. We cannot underestimate the power of this, along with the influence of a lifetime of advertising, which, in the case of freezer pizzas, often features warm Italian kitchens, fresh basil, golden carafes of olive oil and juicy ripe tomatoes, in spite of the fact they were mass-produced in a factory and are about as Italian as Dolmio – which, by the way, is made in Ireland. (We'll examine the history and power of advertising in detail in Chapter 3.)

Of course, an even more 'Mediterranean' approach to my family's meals would be to care so much about food, flavour and health that the very idea of a frozen pizza is an abomination. The mad dash around the shop would never happen, because food would be organized, prioritized, and lovingly cooked at home. For decades now, food companies have heavily reinforced the idea that this way of 'cooking from scratch' is a burden, but maybe we need to unpick this. Such messaging can be powerful, but let's face it, if they can't make us believe that peeling potatoes is a thankless task, they're never going to sell us Smash. In the 1970s and 1980s, adverts for this instant mashed potato, made by Cadbury's, featured aliens watching Earthlings peeling potatoes and laughing at their stupidity. The product, like so many other UPFs, was presented as the future, and sold by the truck load.

Just a few years after the 'Smash Martians' sold us this ultra-processed space food, I got on a plane alone and flew to Lyon, France, to work as an au pair for two months. Aged 17, this was only the second time I had flown, my other excursion being a package holiday to Crete age five. On the flight, I was offered a cold glass of white wine and a beautifully presented langoustine, and this was to be the first bite of a life-changing culinary adventure.

The family I worked for (their name was Dumas – if they are reading, *bonjour et merci!*) lived in a suburban house with a garden, and the next-door house belonged to Mme. Dumas's sister and her family. Every lunchtime and every evening, several courses would be eaten slowly at the shaded outdoor table: fresh bread, saucisson sec, grilled meats, salads, potatoes, cheeses. I had never even tasted bread like it, let alone the rest of it. The sister and her family would arrive with bowls of salads or other contributions, and everyone would gather. It was as if every single meal-time was a party, with the local Beaujolais red wine served chilled from an earthenware pitcher in the fridge. I visited the supermarket many times and was astonished by the chaotic variety – there were even live lobsters! The family food was not complicated, but it was freshly made, savoured slowly, and absolutely never eaten alone. Although I was lucky enough to come from a UK family who cooked and ate together most of the time, I had never before seen this absolute joy and pride in the preparation and sharing of food. The father, who ate every meal with the help of a wooden-handled hunting knife, would talk me through the different cheeses and cured meats with a fierce and patriotic passion. Towards the end of my stay, fluent in French and a stone heavier, they described me as *gourmande*, a uniquely French word that my dictionary told me meant 'greedy', but in fact is a high compliment. In France, to be *gourmande* means to be a 'food lover', delighting in the experience of eating and excited to appreciate each new flavour. A person who would rather fall on their own hunting knife than eat Smash, basically.

The spice of life

That was 1992 – but in the intervening three decades the divide between the British and French tables seems only to have widened. In spite of being our closest neighbour, our eating habits are more similar to the USA, with UK shopping baskets containing around 50 per cent UPF compared with less than 15 per cent in the French trolley. France is not completely free of any issues around changing food choices or obesity, but their laws, for example regarding the ingredients of bread and the percentage of local produce that must be sold in supermarkets, have ensured some of the culture that I experienced with the Dumas family has been protected. The question now is: how can all of us rediscover and protect that culture, because it's not really a 'French' culture, it's actually a fundamentally important part of being human. Researchers at the University of Oxford have shown that the more often people eat together, the more likely they are to feel happy, bonded with each other and with their community, and contented with their life.[10] And yet the same piece of research showed that around a third of UK people's weekday evening meals were being eaten in isolation, with the average adult eating around half their meals alone each week. In the same way that when we eat UPF we are physically missing out on the nutrition that the whole foods we are replacing would have given us, we are also physically missing out on the human connection and pleasure that cooking and eating together can bring. Perhaps we need to channel a bit of Big French Energy in our own lives, insisting on real garlic not the one in the jar, proper bread, decent cheese and everyone round the table?

In truth, the food *chez* Dumas was pretty repetitive: the exact same bread, meats and cheeses each day, every salad dressed in the same homemade dressing. There were no curries and stir-fries, frozen stuff in batter, boxed quiches, pizzas, crisps or ready-made cakes, the usual menu of options we tend to think of as 'variety' – but what do we mean by this? In truth, all of this food, whilst it may have different names and bright, diverse packaging, is made up of very similar ingredients: nearly 60 per cent of our calories come from just three species – rice, maize and wheat – and 75 per cent of the global food supply comes from only twelve plants and five animal species.[11] 'We may think we have a varied diet,' Monica Wilde, author of *The Wilderness Cure*, tells me, 'but there's barely any variation of ingredients. There are many different ways you can process high fructose corn syrup or potatoes, but this doesn't mean you are eating a variety of *species*.' Monica spent a year living entirely from foraged food whilst researching her book and is now heading up the second Wildbiome™ Project, to study what happens to people when they eat a diet entirely made up of wild foods. 'It's a mistake to think of this as a kind of 'pared down' diet, or that you are somehow depriving yourself,' she explains. 'During my year of living off free, wild food in central Scotland, I recorded eating 300 species of plants, 87 species of mushroom, 20 types of seaweed, and 44 species from the animal kingdom. This highly varied diet had a profound impact on my gut microbiome and health.' Monica's Wildbiome™ Project has seen this impact on other participants too: Type 2 diabetes was reversed in one participant, many lost weight and lowered their BMI, several normalized their blood pressure, and species of beneficial bacteria in their guts increased; this research is now widening and ongoing. She says that as well as the health benefits, many people, particularly the young, currently contact her and join her courses with a real desire not just to eat differently, but to live differently. 'I truly believe that humans currently have a profound desire for change, a longing of the heart for connection back to the earth,' she says.

In a culinary journey of a different kind, in 2023 Mike Keen decided to kayak 2,200km solo up the west coast of Greenland, exploring the very opposite of variety by eating an exclusively Inuit diet of mostly fish and sea mammals. A chef by trade, Mike was fascinated by the modern, ultra-processed menu, and what would happen to the body if it went back to absolute basics. I found Mike's story interesting in the context of the pressure so many of us feel to eat a highly varied diet, and I asked him for his take on this: 'when considering what we should be eating now, I always reflect back to how evolution shaped us,' he told me. 'Simple foods, very simple – mostly raw initially, some fermented (some would say rotten) foods and some cooked foods would have been prevalent. And not only simple, but single foods as well. A single animal would often have provided food for several days. The same goes for fish, or a discovery of fruit or honey. It's only relatively recently, evolutionary speaking, that we've been consuming multi-ingredient meals. So for most of our history our bodies would have been dealing with one type of food at a time.'

Part of this, he explains, was through simple necessity, as he discovered in Greenland. 'Before I started, I had visions of setting up camp, finding some driftwood for a fire and getting some good social media footage. In reality, the environment totally dominated and dictated the pace and content of my day. Temperatures of minus 12 degrees Celsius meant that food became purely functional – after a day in freezing cold water and rain, the basic need of warmth and shelter trumped the need for fancier stuff, like taste. Raw meat or fish was barely cooked, if at all – the priority being to get something nutritious inside you as quickly as you could.' Mike subsisted on barely any fruits or vegetables, and ate a diet that would seem, on paper at least, to deprive the body of much-needed nutrition. But something else happened. Throughout his journey his health was monitored closely by researchers and, somewhat extraordinarily, Mike says he became healthier by every metric, including developing a much more diverse gut microbiome. He's now passionate about exploring how 'eating your environment', as he calls it, is optimal for human health, and although he's no longer eating fermented narwhal in a remote Arctic bay, he keeps his UK diet simple: eggs, meat, fish, cheese, and a few berries.

Mike's simple choices may not be desirable or realistic for all of us (in particular the narwhal!), nor would many have the skills or perhaps the desire to subsist off foraged food from the hedgerows, as Monica does. But what these culinary journeys do is force us to re-examine our own choices with fresh eyes. As we look again, we start to unpick some of the myths and lies around the modern food system, which we are told is all about choice, variety and health, but which in fact takes us a long way from all of that and feeds us the same bland, processed starches and sugars each day, dressed up in different shapes and sauces. We can live without all of this. For most of human history we have survived and thrived on diets much more like Monica's, Mike's and the Dumas' – wholefoods, simply prepared and shared. We have had what may seem like 'less', but in many ways this has been 'more' – more connection to nature, to family and to each other, more appreciation of what's on our plates, more mindfulness and gratitude, and often better nutrition and health. UPF companies told us that peeling spuds was a waste of time and offered us an alien future. They hoodwinked us all, but as we will see in the next chapter, there's one group they've really done a number on: women.

3.

A woman's place

The kitchen and promises of liberation

If I show you a picture of a woman in an apron, proudly holding out a cake, you may have a variety of reactions. For some, it's a wholesome image, evoking the comfort of home, of nurturing mothers, and even pride in creative finesse. Others may see it as problematic, regressive, a negative gender stereotype with sexist undertones. For many of us, though, I think it can be both. Most of us have grown up bombarded by mixed messages; home cooking is both a mark of femininity *and* the root of all women's oppression. In this seeming contradiction, UPF manufacturers have found a rich seam they have mined for decades, with advertising and slogans from the 1950s to the present day promising to give us 'home-style' food 'just like momma used to make', whilst offering women time off with 'Swanson night' or 'Dolmio day'. To sell their products, they have to convince us that cookery is simultaneously a wholesome, generous and highly skilled activity, and a complete waste of our time. The kitchen is a prison from which only they can free us: *Liberate Mum: take home some Kentucky Fried Chicken today*, said a KFC ad campaign in the 1970s.

It's hard to know which came first, the chicken or the Egg Beaters: could it be that feminists handed marketing companies an opportunity on a plate when they declared cooking and family life to be domestic slavery? Or did the manufacturers themselves create the idea that time spent in food preparation was completely undesirable, and that their products offered women the freedom they craved? Either way, 'the kitchen' has become so inextricably associated with the dark era of gender inequality that it now stands as metaphor for servitude itself. Eschewing it has become a way to position yourself as empowered: 'I suppose I could have stayed home and baked cookies and had teas, but what I decided to do was to fulfil my profession,' said Hillary Clinton in the early 1990s. 'You'll find me in the studio and not in the kitchen,' sang Lily Allen over two decades later. And another five years after that, Miley Cyrus asked, 'Do people really think that I'm at home in a fucking apron cooking dinner?' Celebrity chef Nigella Lawson subverted this idea in her 2001 manual, *How to Be a Domestic Goddess*: 'sometimes...we don't want to feel like a postmodern, postfeminist, overstretched woman but, rather, a domestic goddess, trailing nutmeggy fumes of baking pie in our languorous wake,' she wrote in the Introduction, but later clarified that the concept was intended to be ironic and that the book was about 'feeling like one rather than actually being one'. To actually *be* one has come to be synonymous with having no other life or ambition; with drudgery.

Your arms – his sink

In 1972, an early subscription offer for the feminist magazine *Spare Rib* was a dishcloth emblazoned with the words: *First you sink into his arms, then your arms end up in his sink.* *Spare Rib* took the decision early on never to include recipes: 'Food preparation was so entwined with the role of the housewife that we consigned it to the bin of history,' wrote one of the magazine's founders, Rosie Boycott, in the *Guardian*.[1] It's easy to see how women had reached boiling point at that historical moment. Although humans had most often had a gender divide in the everyday work of staying alive, with women usually taking care of children and, by extension, food preparation and the home, in the twentieth century this had evolved into something different – a new world of capitalist opportunity, in which men were free to go where they wished, fulfil their ambitions, and make money; and in which women were actively prevented from doing the same.

Practices like the 'Marriage Bar' forced women out of their jobs once wed and were in place from the 1920s until around the late 1940s, after women had joined the workforce as part of the war effort. In some UK institutions, for example the Foreign Service, the Marriage Bar remained until the 1970s and was only made illegal by the Sex Discrimination Act in 1975. It was this Act, too, that enabled women to have their own bank accounts and apply for credit; how hard it must have been to be autonomous without such economic freedom. And one room of the house, the kitchen, became synonymous with this period of patriarchal entitlement and injustice in ways we are yet to fully shake off. Even today the sexist jokes linger – 'Two sugars, luv!' – and some online influencers, from trad wives to Andrew Tate, continue to insist the kitchen is 'a woman's place' and by this they mean that other 'places' – career, sport, travel, adventure, politics, etc. – are men's alone. Ironically, 'trad wives' – women who build huge followings on social media with the message of subservience to their husbands – monetize their content to the max and have economic power and freedom that women of just a few decades ago could only dream of. There's a certain hypocrisy in selling the idea of female subjugation for a sum that you put straight into a bank account that bears your name alone. For most of us, the reality of making dinner is not an Instagrammable affair; it's a task that, rather than being lucrative and rewarding, can feel entirely thankless.

The kitchen and all that takes place there has therefore become a melting pot of ideas and messaging about women's roles and rights, reflecting back our changing cultural norms in each polished saucepan. It is a room full of archetypes – the Good Mother, the Lazy Wife, the Hopeless Husband, the Nurturer, the Seductress, the Wise Grandmother, the Domestic Goddess – and thus an advertiser's dream. One early adopter of this was Daniel Gerber, the maker of one of the first processed baby foods, who spotted the value of selling women not a product in a jar, but a message about themselves and their own lives. Already involved in the business of canned fruit, he moved into the area of fruit purées marketed for babies in 1927 and capitalized on the growing interest of mothers in following the advice of experts when weaning their infants. But the company PR story of how the idea for the product came about has been spun in two different ways over the years.

In the 1990s, the Gerber website told of how it was Mrs Dan Gerber (who is rarely given her own first name of Dorothy) who came up with the idea when she asked her husband to help her strain peas for their baby, a narrative that would have fit well with the enterprising women of that decade. But in the 1930s, an advertorial in a women's magazine told of how Gerber himself had come up with the products, and seemed to aim the story at dads: 'To puzzled fathers of rather young children,' it reads, '...who've had to exchange a charming wife for a tired mother who spends endless hours in the kitchen dutifully scraping, stewing and straining vegetables for your children.' Of course, the advert was not for men to read at all, but women, who were being given a subtle warning about their own likely inadequacy and its potential dire consequences. In both spins of the story, the image of women is co-opted, their desires and insecurities are manipulated, and the product is positioned as their rescuer. Even the baby can be saved by Gerber, because the mother will have more time for him or her. 'For Baby's Sake, Stay Out of the Kitchen!', one 1933 advert proclaimed. All of these tactics were extraordinarily successful and Gerber remains the leading baby food brand in the USA today, although now it belongs to Nestlé.

Add an egg

Like Gerber, most UPF companies promise to help women out of the kitchen whilst at the same time leaning heavily on the mother archetype to sell their products. In the USA in the 1950s, almost every food manufacturer utilized a fictional woman as part of their branding, the most well-known being Betty Crocker, whose brand, part of General Mills, still endures. These entirely made-up women were known in the business as 'live trademarks' and they followed a specific recipe: 'Ideally, the corporate character is a woman, between the ages of 32 and 40, attractive, but not competitively so, mature but youthful-looking, competent yet warm, understanding but not sentimental, interested in the consumer but not involved with her,' explained a trade publication in 1957. Betty Crocker and her invented sisters did everything from appearing in advertising, offering recipes (printed in women's magazines and with a host of branded ingredients, of course!) and even signing off letters to women who wrote to them for domestic advice. In everything they did, the message was clear – these 'mature but youthful-looking' women would show you how to cut corners in the kitchen, winning you praise for being a better woman whilst allowing you to do less of the actual tasks associated with womanhood. Food companies were doing something quite clever here – completely devaluing and undermining traditional cooking methods, on the one hand, and selling themselves as 'mother' on the other, with all the desirable connotations of warmth, nurture and nutrition that this offered.

This messaging was not always straightforward, though. The original early 1950s Betty Crocker cake mix in a packet sold poorly, and the manufacturers turned to the emerging science of psychology to find out why. They called in Edward Bernays, a nephew of Sigmund Freud, who had developed his own application of psychoanalytic theory to marketing and public relations.[2] For example, in the 1920s Bernays had worked for tobacco companies to successfully make cigarette-smoking appealing to women, by creating a campaign that basically told them to smoke instead of eat: 'When tempted by overindulgence, reach for a Lucky instead…and maintain a modern, graceful form.' Drawing on his Uncle Sigmund's ideas about phallic symbols, Bernays also came up with the idea that cigarettes represented masculine power, branding them as 'torches of freedom' and encouraging smoking in public as a way for women to signal their emancipation. Now he tackled cake mix, a brilliant product, or so General Mills thought, because women could make a cake with barely any effort at all. This, said Bernays, was the problem – the product was not selling precisely because it felt too easy, and women felt they were somehow cheating. His solution was to change the recipe and have women 'Add an Egg'. This would not only allow women to feel they were able to take more credit for the finished product, but – at some deeper level – the egg would work as a symbol of life, creation, fertility, and of the woman somehow 'offering up her egg' to her husband. Sales sky-rocketed.

With hindsight, perhaps it was not quite so 'Freudian', but simply that women weren't keen on a cake made entirely from powder. In the hidden reaches of our unconscious minds, we perhaps hold a sense, not of our husband's fertility needs, but of the weight and warmth in our hand of a freshly laid egg from a chicken; and the crackle of tribal fires; and the kneading of dough. Deep down, we know what food truly is, and we know it's not meant to be powdered and in a packet.

Mammy delivers

As well as wearing the archetypal 1950s housewife as a confidence-inspiring costume, food companies have also co-opted the identities of people of colour to sell their products. The most well-known of these is a woman, known as Aunt Jemima, created in 1889 as the trademark for probably the first ever packet mix of 'pancake flour'. The two white men who ran the company, Chris Rutt and Charles G. Underwood, apparently based her on a blackface character one of them had seen in a minstrel show, and drew on the so-called Mammy stereotype to create her look. The Mammy was based on enslaved domestic women, maternal, buxom and often depicted wearing a headscarf. The brand was a huge success, with pancake syrup being added to the range. It soon became a household name and was bought up by Quaker and later by PepsiCo. Like Betty Crocker, real women, most notably the formerly enslaved woman Nancy Green, were employed to play the role of Aunt Jemima at trade shows, cooking pancakes and telling romanticized stories of a Deep South that portrayed black and white people living in harmony. Over the decades, Aunt Jemima's look was changed, and by the late 1980s she had lost her headscarf, slimmed down and been given gold earrings. In 2020, following the murder of George Floyd, Quaker and its parent company, PepsiCo, announced they would discontinue the brand, and by June 2021 the name, as well as the image, had been replaced with 'Pearl Milling Company'.

Aunt Jemima was not the only woman of colour to be used to sell food products. Mrs. Butterworth's was another brand of pancake syrup that came in a bottle said by some to be shaped as a maid or Mammy stereotype. In 2020 the brand owner, Conagra, announced it would review the bottle design, but to date it remains unchanged. Black men have also been used as trademarks, the most well-known being Uncle Ben's rice, rebranded to Ben's Rice in 2020. During slavery and Jim Crow, black people were deemed unworthy of the title of Mr or Mrs, and instead addressed as Uncle and Aunt, so, as with Aunt Jemima, it was implied that Uncle Ben was serving you your packet rice. Both slaves and housewives make for good branding in UPF, it seems, since the images of both align with products that perform menial tasks for you whilst allowing you to recline in your state of privilege. Meanwhile, the rich white men behind the brands are the least likely to be negatively impacted by UPF, whilst women and black people are specifically targeted in their marketing. One study in 2022 found that US food companies disproportionately market unhealthy food and drink, including candy, sodas, snacks and fast food, to black and Hispanic children, teens and adults.[3] Other studies have had similar findings, with one revealing that black children were exposed to 50 per cent more fast-food adverts than their white peers.[4]

Influential puppets

The stratospheric rise of the most popular live trademark, Betty Crocker, was due to two colliding factors, both gifts to the marketing department at her company, General Mills: the advent of radio, and an absolute dearth of restrictions for advertising. Whereas now we expect transparency from broadcasters and want to know when we are being educated and informed, and when we are being sold to, back in the mid-twentieth century this was completely unregulated. Crocker – who, let's not forget, wasn't actually a real person at all – was first heard on the radio as early as the 1920s, and for several decades she dispensed cooking advice that absolutely always incorporated numerous mentions of General Mills products. On radio, this worked brilliantly, and Crocker's persona was authoritative – powerful, even. But as technology moved towards television, it became harder for her to keep her appeal – the packaged cakes that required no effort didn't make for very interesting viewing. Crocker was replaced by a new generation of TV cooks who were real and genuine women, most notably Julia Child, whose programmes from the 1960s you can still watch on YouTube, sleeves rolled up, practically attired, and passionate about French cooking.

One senses that Julia Child was the moment when food companies lost control of the airwaves, a control that today they are perhaps more easily able to regain. In 2023, an investigation by the *Washington Post* revealed that American Beverage Association, a trade group representing Coca-Cola and PepsiCo, were reportedly paying TikTok and Instagram influencers to counter negative press after the WHO named the artificial sweetener aspartame as 'possibly carcinogenic'.[5] These influencers, who were all female dieticians with huge online followings, used the hashtag #*safetyofaspartame* to tell their followers that health concerns about drinking soda were overblown.

Interestingly, dietician is a largely female profession, it's thought perhaps because it has its roots in both nursing and in home economics, the latter being one of the first subjects women were allowed to major in at college. The *Washington Post* investigation also found that other dietician influencers – always female – were creating posts about the benefits of sugary food like doughnuts and sweets as part of paid partnerships with the Canadian Sugar Institute. The regulatory body of dieticians in the USA, the Academy of Nutrition and Dietetics (AND) (see also page 77), whose members are almost entirely female, does have a code of ethics that warns that conflicts of interest should be disclosed. However, the AND arguably has such a conflict itself, given that the Academy has accepted millions of dollars in donations from leading UPF companies like Coca-Cola, PepsiCo and Nestlé, and two of their main sponsors are American Beverage Association and Tate & Lyle. It would seem that while food companies have lost their live trademarks, they are still using women as puppets whenever and wherever possible.

Big skinny lies

Today, food marketing has diversified, with the current emphasis on 'healthy' or 'sustainable' food in 'recyclable' packaging, rather than on cheating your way to housewifery gold. But the world of food is still gendered, as you'll know if you've been to a barbeque recently, where the men inevitably grill the meat as the women usually make the salads. Food advertising now aims some products exclusively at men – think Yorkie bars with the slogans *It's not for girls* and *King size not queen size*, and those 'grab bags' of beefy crisps, with the implication that only men are permitted to have big appetites. Just like Gerber's letter to 'puzzled fathers', these adverts carry a message to women, too, essentially: 'be smaller'. This is reinforced by the multitude of products claiming to help us achieve this goal – think most yoghurts and, well, anything that claims to be 'low fat' or 'diet'. Here's a short story that says so much: 'Coke Zero' is an almost identical recipe to 'Diet Coke', but was created specifically to appeal to men. So the idea that 'diet' products are 'only for girls' is clearly deeply engrained, as is the wholesale avoidance of perceived 'women's products' by men. Misogyny, it seems, is alive and well, even in the fizzy drinks aisle.

The more of these 'health claims' on women's products, the more likely the product is to be UPF. 'Low fat' or 'fat free' yoghurt, for example, is often very high in sugar and can contain other ingredients like gums and starches to thicken and improve the texture, as well as artificial sweeteners like aspartame. 'Low calorie' ice cream is also packed with sweeteners, emulsifiers, starches and thickening gums, as well as mono- and diglycerides of fatty acids, which contain trans fats. Trans fats became popular in the 1980s when the idea of a low-fat diet first took off, with campaigners insisting that animal fats in food were unhealthy and better replaced with vegetable oils. The food industry responded by hydrogenating the oil so that it had a longer shelf-life and was thicker and more solid, making it ideal to bulk up foods cheaply whilst making their health claims. Within a decade, however, it became clear that these trans fats were in fact damaging to humans, causing increased cholesterol and heart disease. Trans fats are now banned in several countries, including the USA, but they are not banned the UK – and you'll find them on labels in the form of hydrogenated oils, partially hydrogenated oils, and mono- and diglycerides of fatty acids, very often in products with words like, 'diet', 'halo', 'go ahead', 'low fat', 'light', 'lite', 'no added sugar', 'fat free', 'low calorie' and even 'skinny' on the front of the pack.

In fact, the use of the word 'skinny' on products has mushroomed recently, with everyone from This Is Skinny Cocktails to Skinny Dream chocolate bars to The Skinny Cookie Company using it in their branding. It's interesting how this word, which can mean scrawny, gaunt or emaciated, has come to be associated with foods making health claims, at a time when we are all supposed to be more aware of both the importance of body positivity and the prevalence of eating disorders. Clearly by putting 'skinny' front and centre on packaging, food companies are particularly trying to appeal to women and girls, and are suggesting – two decades after Kate Moss was slated for saying that 'nothing tastes as good as skinny feels' – that 'skinny' is still very much aspirational for women, regardless of culture, background or age. This is reflected on the catwalk: research from *Vogue* has found that the use of plus-sized models is on the wane, with 95.6 per cent of looks being worn by US sizes zero to four in the major fashion weeks of 2023;[6] and at the same time the use of weight-loss drugs like Ozempic and Wegovy rapidly expands.

In 2024 one UPF company, The Skinny Food Company (owned by the similarly emotively named Not Guilty Food Company), had its advert banned by the Advertising Standards Authority as 'irresponsible'.[7] The advert, a reel posted by the influencer Katie Price on Instagram, featured her meals over the course of the day, all containing 'Skinny' products and adding up to a total of just 755 calories – for context, the recommended daily calorie intake for an adult woman is 2,000. Videos like Price's, with the hashtag #whatIeatinaday, are a draw for young people with eating disorders, perpetuating a damaging cycle of comparison and guilt, says Marcelle Rose, eating disorder specialist and author of *The Binge Freedom Method*™. 'This content often glorifies overly restrictive eating habits, validating myths about food, portion sizes, and calorie intake that can morph into deeply ingrained beliefs. By presenting an unrealistic ideal of what a day's eating 'should' look like, this content can act as a potent trigger. For someone with anorexia, it reinforces the notion that extreme calorie restriction is not only acceptable but aspirational, further entrenching the disorder and hindering recovery.' I asked Marcelle for her thoughts on orthorexia – a newly proposed category of eating disorder in which the sufferer becomes too focused on 'eating healthy' or 'eating clean'. Could conversations about ultra-processed food be potentially damaging to women and girls, creating anxiety? 'Fundamentally, yes,' says Marcelle. 'The messaging around UPFs has the potential to intensify feelings of guilt or fear around certain foods. This risk also applies to individuals dealing with other forms of disordered eating, as overly restrictive messages about food can exacerbate current struggles or cause past eating disorders to resurface.' I wondered, too, about the potential for food companies to seize upon this message, though, and convince us that 'healthy eating can be dangerous'. Marcelle agreed: 'Food companies may capitalize on the idea that 'you can eat too healthily' as a marketing tactic. We need to advocate for transparent, science-based messaging that encourages flexibility and balanced, mindful eating habits.'

The wolf is not grandma

Food companies have consistently told us their products offer freedom from domestic work, but has this happened? Throughout every decade since Betty Crocker first took to the airwaves in 1924, women have continued to carry the responsibility for food shopping, meal planning and food preparation. Even today, the people doing the food shopping are still mostly women – in the UK nearly 80% of women say they have the primary responsibility for this,[8] and in the USA the figures are similar.[9] Twenty-first-century women are arguably the most over-loaded females who have ever lived – work, relationships, family – the myth of 'having it all' has ended up with the endless struggle of the juggle, in which most of us are still doing much more in the house than men, and having considerably less leisure time (around five hours less, according to the Office for National Statistics (ONS)). A poll from YouGov in February 2020 found that household tasks were hugely disproportionately shared, with UK women up to six times more likely than men to say that only they clean the bathroom and do the laundry.[10] Women are also more likely to be the ones doing jobs such as dusting and polishing surfaces, with over half of women stating that they alone do these jobs. On top of this we have the expectations and pressure of jobs and careers, as well as the increasingly well-documented 'mental load' – that phenomenon where we find we are the ones who are carrying so much more in our heads: remembering and organizing birthdays, keeping the social calendar, the kids' shoe sizes, who needs a dental appointment and when and, of course, what's for dinner. If UPF was supposed to make women's lives easier, this appears to have failed spectacularly.

It's clear that food companies have sold us an awful lot of lies. If they were a fairy-tale character, they would be the Wolf in *Little Red Riding Hood*, sitting in the bed wearing Grandma's frilly bonnet and trying to trick us into seeing them as a kindly old dear when in fact they're keen to eat us whole. They've told us we have to choose between liberation and the kitchen, as if it isn't entirely possible to have both. They've taken our millennial-old human need for the deep satisfaction, and even the feeling of being loved and nurtured that being 'cooked for' can provide, and they've sold us the fake version, packaged up in plastic and rammed full of xanthan gum and maltodextrin. They've used our images in their promises of freedom whilst tying us to poor health and obesity. They've offered us the gift of extra time, but they're part of the same capitalist world that sees us all working longer and longer hours and sharing less and less human connection. They have worn the mask of the maternal in order to sell more cake mix but underneath they are, and have always been, the face of patriarchal greed. Dressed up as Betty Crocker, they are shafting us all; wreaking damage on human health and wellbeing, from our very first breath.

4.

Start them young

How the UPF industry exploits mothers and children

When my first child was born I was one of those mums who turned parenting into an academic project. Turning things into an academic project was something I knew how to do; mothering was not. So I read books. The idea that there was a correct path to follow with its own 'how to' manual made me feel stable during what is arguably the most destabilizing transition a woman will ever experience. At the time I was also a practising therapist, working with a variety of different clients, including children in foster care with histories of abuse and neglect. I knew a lot about child development, attachment, bonding, and what can happen when love, stability and the positive unconditional regard of someone who will never let you down are not in place. So I think, with my professional background, and all the parenting books I had read, and all the thinking I did about how to give my three babies the best chance to have a good, loving relationship with others and with themselves, I probably did an OK job. I filled my kids with a healthy balance of love and boundaries, and I dished up a childhood packed with cuddles, books, nature, music and play. Their emotional and psychological start in life was, to paraphrase the psychiatrist Donald Winnicott, 100 per cent 'good enough'.

But I got something completely wrong. With all the love I poured into them morning, noon and night, I barely gave a thought to food and nutrition. This is particularly ironic, considering I breastfed them all until they were around four years old (and buckle up, because we're going to come to breastfeeding later in this chapter). But when it came to the food I offered them as they were weaned onto solids, I think I probably really messed up. I've thought about this a lot and I think that at least part of the reason is because two ideas collided in my head and merged into a very overflowing UPF biscuit tin. The first idea came from my therapy background and, put simply, it was along the lines of, 'don't make food an issue of control'. Having worked with a few young people with eating disorders, I felt like a really laid-back attitude to food was the best plan. No 'finish what's on your plate or you won't get dessert', no labelling foods as 'good' or 'naughty', no offering sweets as rewards or treats, etc. I wanted to avoid any power games around the dinner table and let my kids make autonomous choices about what they ate, and I also didn't want to attach values to particular foods, for example that cake is 'sinful'. As a *gourmande* myself (see page 52), I wanted them to develop a love and a passion for food, and having sat and held space for young girls with anorexia, I wanted them to learn not so much that 'broccoli is good for me' but that 'eating is good for me'. Because it really is, right? Cooking and sharing and eating food is one of the great pleasures of life, isn't it? And if you don't eat, you die, therefore eating is good for you. And all food is good…errr…hmmm…this is where my thinking merged into the second idea, and fell apart a bit.

Because the second idea was basically, 'all food is good for you'. And I think I felt like this was the right overall message to give them – that there are no bad foods, and that everything is okay as part of a balanced diet. In fact, I believed that myself. But not only is this idea shaky at best, it was almost certainly planted in my mind – and in the minds of my parents before me and indeed many of you reading this now – by those with a vested interest in me purchasing and eating their ultra-processed products. When UPF was in its infancy in the 1970s, environmentalists and activists protested. Their message, that food-like items whipped up in factories and filled with additives were not only bad for us and the planet but weren't even food at all, was a direct threat to the profits of major food companies. During the 1970s and 1980s, these companies made it their business to counter this message: they employed doctors, scientists and nutritionists to vigorously promote everything from the health benefits of sugar to the equivalence of the potato chip to broccoli, with statements like, 'when eaten with your lunchtime sandwich, (crisps) add vegetable nutrition to help balance the meal'.[1] Industry fact sheets were put out via the American Dietetic Association (ADA), hammering home the message that *all* foods are healthy foods as part of a balanced diet. In fact, the ADA – now called the Academy of Nutrition and Dietetics – still takes this line in its most recent position statement: *'It is the position of the Academy of Nutrition and Dietetics that the total diet or overall pattern of food eaten is the most important focus of healthy eating. All foods can fit within this pattern if consumed in moderation with appropriate portion size and combined with physical activity. The Academy strives to communicate healthy eating messages that emphasize a balance of food and beverages within energy needs, rather than any one food or meal.'*[2]

This 'total diet' approach – which could have been written by me when I was weaning my kids – sounds eminently sensible and seems to come from a highly reputable source. Visit the Academy of Nutrition and Dietetics website and it tells you that it is 'the world's largest organization of food and nutrition professionals', and it does look like a huge database of nutrition specialists, with plenty of stock images of broccoli and resources about how to 'eat right'. But in 2015 its corporate sponsors included Coca-Cola, PepsiCo, General Mills, Kellogg's and Unilever.[3] And in this year, and in their most recent annual reports for 2021[4] and 2022[5] their biggest 'premier sponsor' was Abbott, makers of Similac Infant Formula Milk.

A company funded in this way has a vested interest in making sure that none of us writes off certain foods as 'junk' and leaves them out of our shopping trolley. The message that 'there are no bad foods' and 'everything is part of a balanced diet' is a gift to anyone who has a UPF to sell. And here I am, a mum in the UK, and that message filtered through to me loud and clear, skewing my own choices when I chose not only my own diet, but the items I would feed to my children. If I could go back and again be responsible for introducing three brand-new, box-fresh humans to solid food, I would get a red pen out and add to the message like this: 'Everything is part of a balanced diet BUT THAT MEANS ACTUAL FOOD NOT UPF!' The Academy of Nutrition and Dietetics might disagree with me, though – amazingly, in spite of hundreds of articles on its website, not one mentions the term 'ultra-processed'. There is just one piece about 'processed food', just one! And it tells us that, although this type of food has a bad reputation, 'it might be a surprise to learn that whole-wheat bread, homemade soup or a chopped apple also are processed foods'.[6] It's hard to believe that an organization responsible for dietary advice across America doesn't know what it is doing here – muddling the definition of 'processing' as if slicing a piece of fruit in any way changes its nutritional qualities. No wonder some people are confused about the definition of UPF, if they are being told that homemade soup is in the same category as 'drive-thru hamburgers'.

The British Nutrition Foundation (BNF) also blurs the lines in its May 2024 position statement, telling us that the Nova definition is 'broad' and that 'the definition of UPF can also include foods such as sliced wholemeal bread and lower sugar wholegrain breakfast cereals which can contribute to an affordable healthy, balanced diet'.[7] But you could argue that the BNF also has a vested interest in the 'everything is fine as part of a balanced diet' message, given that its funding comes from every major UK supermarket along with a long list of major corporations, including Kellogg's, Coca-Cola, Greggs, Costa, Danone, Nestlé and McDonald's.[8] Of course, the Scientific Advisory Committee on Nutrition (SACN) – a UK government body – agrees with the BNF that UPF is not clearly defined and should not be included in national dietary guidelines. But the SACN's sixteen committee members have some declared interests: five are members of the American Society of Nutrition, a US dietary organization that is funded by Mars, Nestlé and Mondelēz; two have financial relationships with the British Nutrition Foundation; one is a shareholder in Sainsbury's; one is a paid consultant for several food and fizzy drink companies, including Tate & Lyle; two are funded by UPF giant Danone; one is on the council of the Nestlé Foundation for the Study of Problems of Nutrition in the World; one is a former employee and current shareholder in Unilever.[9]

We all like to think we have freedom of thought and freedom of choice, especially when it comes to fundamental decisions that might have long-lasting consequences, such as the way we feed our children. My approach with my kids was to offer them 'everything' and let them enjoy 'all food'. But I didn't realize how much the messaging of global food companies might be influencing my thinking, convincing me that, as long as my kids were getting roughly the right nutrition, it didn't really matter what form that nutrition was taking. Too late now, I've come to understand that there's a difference between 'nutrition' and 'nourishment', a difference between a 'balanced diet' and a diet that includes UPF. If I had a magic wand, I'd wave it over my kitchen circa 2010 and remove the UPF biscuits and cakes, the chocolatey breakfast cereals, the frozen pizza and chicken nuggets, the flavoured yoghurts, and the sugar-free squash. Because even though I'm a good cook, and so is their dad, and we offered up plenty of homemade meals, I genuinely believed that these UPF foods weren't a problem, as long as there was some broccoli and carrots in the mix as well. I guess I even thought that some of them were staples of a happy, fun childhood. Essentially, in spite of my passion for breastfeeding, I'd fallen for a nutritional message beloved of formula companies: stuff made in a factory is not much different from stuff you can make yourself, and the main thing is that everyone has a bellyful of roughly the right amount of calories and nutrition each day – in other words, 'fed is best'.

Fed is best

Quite a few people have asked me if I'm going to 'go there' with breastfeeding and formula in this book, and yes, I am. Having written about the topic many times over the years, I do know how divisive it can be, but I don't think this means we should be afraid of discussing it. I write from a place of absolute respect and support for every single woman and her choices, and also from the perspective that it's too important a topic to be off-limits. It would be remiss to write a book about UPF and women without being brave enough to mention the elephant in the room: formula milk is ultra-processed. It is a powder made by a process of industrial-level dry blending or spray-drying and may contain oils, including palm oil, and additives, such as emulsifiers. It is different from breast milk, which is a live substance, tailormade for the baby, dynamically changing in response to their needs.

However, it's important to acknowledge just how painful this subject can be if you are a woman whose breastfeeding experience was difficult. We know that, in the UK for example, around 80 per cent of women say they stopped breastfeeding before they wanted to.[10] I know from experience of talking to many such women that they very often blame themselves and feel their bodies were somehow not up to the task. In fact, a physical inability to breastfeed is very rare, and it's much more likely to be lack of support or bad advice that was actually the cause of their struggles. Ultimately, though, whether it was your body or the system that let you down, the grief that many women feel is still the same, and I have no desire to add to those difficult feelings. For this reason, this chapter is not focused on individual women's breastfeeding stories and experiences, but instead shines a spotlight on the tactics of the formula companies and explores how they mirror those of the manufacturers of other forms of UPF (and they are often the same companies, of course – Danone makes Cow & Gate and Aptamil; Nestlé makes SMA).

Although I breastfed my children, the tactics of UPF companies derailed my thinking when I came to wean them and I now regret some of the foods that have been part of their childhood. I feel really bad that my choices have potentially damaged their health in some way, when all I want for them is the absolute best. But, although we can make changes now and for the future, it's too late to change the past. It's too late for many of us to change how we fed our kids, or how we were fed as kids, or how we've been feeding ourselves – and contemplating this can be painful, causing us to feel defensive, or bad, or both. But what if we think about the wisdom we've gained from our mistakes? What if we shift our focus onto future women and think about what, in an ideal world, we want for them? If the answer to that is 'freedom of choice', then we need to spend a bit of time unpicking how our choices are informed, and whether or not they're really, truly 'free'. Because just as I 'freely chose' to dish up chicken nuggets to my kids and spoon-feed them from jars of 'baby food', not realizing that my choices were informed by subtle but powerful messages from the food industry, women from all parts of the world who feed their babies formula are often under the same sway.

When we use the term 'infant formula' we are arguably already participating in the marketing of a product. Since humans began to try to make a marketable substance that would feed babies safely, around the mid-nineteenth century, there has been a concerted effort to give this process an air of 'science'. Hence we have 'formula' and brand names like 'Similac' (similar to lactation), 'Aptamil', 'Enfamil' and SMA (simulated milk adapted). Nobody is branding powdered baby milk 'Boobylicious' or 'Teatily Terrific' – it just wouldn't inspire the same confidence. Likewise, the packaging of formula is also carefully designed to make parents feel they are purchasing something high standard and safe, with gold lettering and words like 'advanced', 'healthy' and 'pro', alongside claims of being 'comforting' for colic, of nutritional benefits or of impact on IQ or baby's sleep. These claims vary from country to country depending on how tightly regulated their packaging is: the looser the regulation, the wider the claims.

Although people had been working on various recipes to try and replicate breast milk commercially for a while, formula didn't really get off the ground until the 1950s, and it's no coincidence that demand began to soar around the same time that birth moved into hospitals and women's post-natal experience began to be 'managed' by well-meaning helpers. Babies were removed from their mothers and brought to them when the clock, rather than the baby, dictated; women were made to wash their nipples before and after feeds; babies were weighed with scrutiny and 'topped up' after strictly timed breastfeeding sessions. All of this interferes with the natural and hormonal process of breastfeeding, which relies on physical contact with the baby and nursing on demand in order to stimulate supply. The interference can also lead to engorgement, poor latch, pain and mastitis and 'not enough milk' – all of which make formula either appealing or necessary. In 2024, we have still not moved fully away from these practices and continue to disrupt the mother-infant relationship in a variety of ways whilst simultaneously puzzling over why breastfeeding is beset with difficulties. The formula industry has come to rely on those difficulties, and to work hard and unscrupulously to exacerbate them.

Profit over ethics

During the same post-war decades that saw the advent of these counter-productive post-natal practices, Nestlé was busy in Africa and Asia, where it spotted a new market. Through aggressive advertising campaigns, it convinced mothers that this new type of feeding was scientific, futuristic and safe, even employing starchily uniformed 'milk nurses' – but they weren't nurses at all, they were saleswomen.[11] These 'nurses' told mothers that breastfeeding was best, but then went on to explain just how complicated the nutrition of their breastfed baby would be, telling them, for example, of the vitamins, cereals and freshly made fruit juices they would have to offer as supplements. Formula was then offered as a much simpler alternative. Convinced to choose this new type of milk, women's breast-milk supply would then dry up, making them completely dependent on Nestlé's product, whatever the cost, to keep their baby alive.[12]

Into an environment with an unreliable supply of clean water and limited resources and support, Nestlé sold a product that had to be made correctly if babies' lives were not to be put at risk. Needless to say, many thousands of babies died from what became known as 'commerciogenic malnutrition' or 'bottle baby disease'. News of this situation spread during the 1970s, and in 1978 Nestlé and other milk companies were called to testify to Congress in the USA, where they struggled to defend their ethics. As a result, many people began to boycott Nestlé, and still do to this day. In 1981, an international code for formula marketing was developed by the World Health Organization, known as 'the WHO Code', setting new standards for all formula companies to hopefully follow. Although not law, this code was adopted in many countries to some degree.

At a moment in history when such companies, in particular Nestlé, could have reflected on their actions with shame, they chose instead to focus on ways to get around this new set of guidelines. Suddenly restricted from being allowed to advertise milk for babies from birth to six months, Nestlé invented a whole new, completely unnecessary product just to circumvent the rules – 'Follow-on Milk', marketed for babies from six to twelve months.[13] A bit of breastfeeding background: it's widely agreed that a formula-fed baby needs formula milk for the first year, after which they can have cow's milk. There is absolutely no need for 'follow-on milk' – they can drink the same infant formula for the first twelve months. In fact, this is probably better as some follow-on milks tend to be high in sugar; a recent report from First Steps Nutrition Trust in the UK has revealed that some toddler milks contain more sugar than a chocolate milkshake.[14] But by creating this product, formula companies were able to advertise. They use near-identical packaging and branding for their follow-on milks, and the equally unnecessary 'Toddler Milk' and 'Growing-up Milk', with the sole purpose of getting their brand in front of you. Any baby drinking formula beyond the age of one is consuming unnecessary UPF, completely surplus to their nutritional requirements. In their follow-on milk adverts, breastfeeding is often mentioned, ensuring that the association is made in people's minds between these two 'products', and viewers are also often pointed to formula company websites, which contain 'helpful' resources that are all about…breastfeeding? Surprising? Why would they want to help women breastfeed? Well of course, in an industry whose $55 billion a year revenue depends on you *not* breastfeeding, they don't.

In the UK, and in many other countries where formula milk has become the norm, there is a diabolical lack of funding into feeding support for new mothers. According to the last

Infant Feeding Survey in the UK, for example, over 80 per cent initiate breastfeeding at birth, but by six weeks post-partum, in England only 24 per cent are exclusively breastfeeding – and this number is even lower in Wales (17 per cent) and Northern Ireland (13 per cent).[15] Whilst there are pockets of good support and many brilliant individual practitioners, women often struggle to find face-to-face help and accurate information, turning to Google when in the past they may have turned to older relatives and friends.

Let's look at the current breastfeeding page on the Aptamil UK website, which many of these women may find in their search for help and information.[16] It's written by a well-known TV doctor, and it starts by telling us how great breastfeeding is for both woman and baby. But in the first paragraph it opens by telling us that Aptamil's website will help with 'common breastfeeding problems' and reminds women not to put 'too much pressure' on themselves, and maybe try 'expressing and storing milk when you have the energy, so you can continue breastfeeding as soon as you can'. Hmm, it's already sounding like breastfeeding is going to be quite tiring, stressful and tricky, isn't it? The next section tells women how important their diet will be when they are breastfeeding, and what foods they will have to include or avoid. But in fact, all the evidence shows that lactation is a highly efficient process and that the vital nutrients in breast milk are not affected by diet, or even by famine.[17] In times of extreme malnutrition, the mother's nutrient reserves are mobilised to ensure that breast milk quality is not compromised, and although this will eventually impact the mother's health, it does serve to illustrate that making ordinary women who are not in a survival situation feel anxious about their diets is completely unnecessary. Telling women they need to eat or cut out particular foods, especially post-pregnant women who are already longing for a juicy rare steak and a pint of beer, plants another seed of doubt. Then the next section on the Aptamil page is, 'Breastfeeding Problems'. You get the idea.

Rather like many UPF manufacturers, formula companies also position themselves as feminist (and breastfeeding advocates, therefore, as holding women back), with one 2015 advertising campaign from Similac evoking the 'sisterhood of motherhood' and positioning breastfeeding advocacy as trivial and divisive.[18] Here again is the key UPF strategy of telling women they have a problem and that their product is the solution; for new mums, crying and sleeping offer themselves up on a plate as problems that need to be urgently solved. At a 2017 international trade event, the CEO of an Irish nutrition company said that formula milk wasn't necessarily about the ingredients: 'What we are selling is actually sleep...If the baby doesn't sleep for three nights and the mother is exhausted, the mother will change the infant formula. So that's what we're selling.'[19] Another CEO added that they were also selling 'peace of mind'.

One way formula companies achieve this is by getting health professionals on board, with a long history of advertising in professional journals and sponsoring their events. To name just one example, the March 2024 conference of the *British Journal of Midwifery* was sponsored by Aptamil, Kendamil and Nestlé, with each of the three having a forty-minute slot at the one-day meeting. Formula companies now also have technology at their disposal, with the ability to know if you're pregnant or just interested in infant feeding from your social media posts, and perhaps even know when you are awake at 3 a.m. and struggling with your newborn. Some women actively don't want to breastfeed, and it's absolutely their right to choose. Many women do want to breastfeed but end their breastfeeding journey sooner than they had wished to, often feeling like they have failed or that their bodies have let them down. It's wrong that they should have to feel this way, when what is actually to blame is a culture that is highly unsupportive of breastfeeding, constantly fuelled in ever more innovative ways by the companies whose sales success depends entirely on breastfeeding failure.[20]

The unscrupulous tactics of formula companies in low- and middle-income countries continue to this day. During the Covid-19 pandemic, free samples of formula were given out to communities in Africa under lockdown, alongside claims of protection from Covid via formula,[21] or the (false) risk of breastfeeding whilst infected.[22] In 2018, Danone was accused of misleading women with an advertising campaign in Turkey that warned mothers they might not be making enough milk: 'Your baby needs at least 500ml milk per day. If your breast milk is not enough, give Aptamil formula to support your baby's immune system', their advert claimed.[23] But perhaps there is an unconscious racism inherent in the idea that only poor, black and brown women's breastfeeding rates can be affected by these unprincipled practices, whereas in the higher income West we are not so easily influenced and use formula out of 'choice'. By the same token, it is somehow more acceptable to talk about improving breastfeeding rates in low-income countries, whilst in the West the topic is fraught with difficulty, with the constant refrain of 'fed is best' and even calls to remove the WHO Code entirely by those who see it as a barrier to women's freedom. Just as UPF companies' sales relied on my thinking that a jar of baby food was just as nutritious for my baby as homemade spaghetti sauce, formula companies benefit from any discussion of the benefits of breastfeeding being potentially divisive. Let's not keep falling into that trap.

UPF from day one

In the context of this book it's also worth noting that using formula normalizes UPF, even in families who breastfeed. It encourages us to put our ultimate trust in 'food from a packet' right from birth and carries the message that such food is 'equivalent' – possibly even superior – to food made in more natural ways. It undermines trust in nature herself. In those of us who are fed it – and I was one – it trains the palate to expect bland conformity: where every mouthful of formula tastes the same, breast milk is constantly changing, reflecting the foods a mother eats in the same way that the flavour of her amniotic fluid did in utero.[24] And it develops consumer trust in the brands and 'foods in plastic' that continue to be offered in every supermarket aisle as a child is weaned onto 'solids'.

When my first child reached six months, I was slightly terrified of the weaning process and had no idea what to give her. Perhaps picking up on my new mum anxiety, she treated food pretty sceptically, which only fed my worries. It felt somehow easier to offer her little packs of 'melty carrot puffs' or spaghetti from a jar (we even had a song about that!). And although by the time her sister was born I'd got a bit more confident and tried out 'baby-led weaning' (a system where you offer mainly the same foods as you are eating yourself, and let the baby use their hands to feed themselves), I still offered fromage frais, pouches of fruit purée that she could hold and suck, and a fair amount of what is jokingly called 'freezer tapas', a.k.a fish fingers, nuggets and chips. My third and final baby was the one with all the allergies, so he got plenty of UPF too in the form of 'dairy-free' yoghurts, vegan margarine, and treats in the form of the cheapest supermarket biscuits because these are usually made without butter. It's only mildly comforting to know that I'm not alone – according to the First Steps Nutrition Trust, only 6 per cent of UK parents with a youngest child aged one year did not buy any commercial baby food or drinks.[25]

Food marketed as being specifically for babies and children in the UK is subject to fairly strict regulation, meaning that often, from the ingredients list alone, you would perhaps not assess them as UPF. However, these types of food are the next step on the UPF journey: they are often high in sugar, bland and predictable in texture and taste, easy to over-consume either because of texture or the encouragement to suck them from a pouch, and offering none of the multi-sensory experience of food that is so vital in early development in order for children to learn about food preparation, variety, texture and taste. Then there are other UPFs, that don't say anywhere on the packaging that they are for children but that feature favourite TV characters, which are less regulated and therefore often contain more additives. The market for 'finger food' for toddlers is growing rapidly, encouraging children into the habit of snacking from an early age, often with products that are marketed as 'healthy' but which highly resemble unhealthy adult snacks, such as UPF crisps, sweets and biscuits. Presumably this imitation is an intentional tactic, with the UPF companies hoping to create customers for life.

And it's working. Between the ages of two and five, UPF is thought to make up around two-thirds of the average child's diet in both the UK and USA: the habits are in place. This trend seems to be largely universal, although in the UK researchers found young people from disadvantaged backgrounds consumed the highest amount, and that white children consumed more UPF than those from other ethnicities.[26] UPF consumption is reinforced at school, where around two-thirds of the calories are currently coming from UPF in the average school dinner, and a whopping 70 per cent UPF in the average packed lunch.[27] Trust me, I've been there, bunging in all the different packets in the mad morning rush – the Fruit Winders ('one of your five a day'), the fromage frais ('made with calcium for stronger bones'), the crisps ('added vegetable nutrition to balance the meal'?!) – and who wants to be the parent who says 'No' and whose kid feels different or left out? It's so convenient, and the marketing may even convince us we are doing our children a favour, but we're really not. In many UK schools, including the one my own kids attended, children brought in packets of sweets to distribute on their birthday, and with over thirty-five kids in the class, this meant a bag of candy roughly once a week. Not only do all these choices normalize UPF for our kids from such a young age, setting the trajectory of their palates and eating patterns, they also have implications for their long-term health. These trends continue, with adolescents consuming the highest levels of UPF – it's pretty much baked in to our thinking that teenagers will be happiest when given fast food, frozen pizzas and fizzy drinks, isn't it? Food companies spend billions marketing to this age group, with over 90 per cent of their entire budget being spent on advertising sugary drinks and fast food, with ever-growing opportunities now to reach young people directly while they are gaming or online.[28]

We can no longer excuse ourselves for conceptualizing sweets, sodas and junk food as 'kids' food' or even a 'treat'. There are now several good-quality studies that show a clear link between childhood UPF consumption and childhood obesity, as well as the potential for bodily growth restriction, probably due to the lost nutrients in the diet from whole foods displaced by UPF.[29] Around 20–30 per cent of UK four- to five-year-olds are living with obesity and overweight, putting them at increased risk of a lifetime of health problems. According to the World Health Organization, obese and overweight children are likely to stay obese into adulthood and to be at higher risk of developing noncommunicable diseases like diabetes and cardiovascular disease from a younger age.[30] A Spanish study in May 2024 looked at children between the ages of three and six years and found that higher UPF consumption was associated with higher BMI, larger waist circumference, greater fat levels and higher blood sugar, putting them at risk of poor heart health and diabetes.[31]

This follows other studies, including one that found that children consuming higher UPF at age three have higher cholesterol by age six.[32] Another study has found a link between higher UPF consumption and dental caries in children,[33] and as our understanding of the microbiome grows, we can no longer treat the mouth and teeth as something separate from the gut, or indeed from the brain and mental health. Researchers in 2022 found a direct association between high consumption of UPF and low mood, emotional distress and behavioural problems in adolescents,[34] whilst another study the following year found that Spanish adolescents who consumed UPFs regularly were more likely to have mood and anxiety problems.[35] UPF displaces healthy food from the diet: in a cross-sectional study published in the *British Medical Journal* in 2022, higher fruit and vegetable consumption in secondary school children was significantly associated with higher mental wellbeing.[36] Behavioural issues can also be impacted by what we eat: there is increasing attention being paid to the impact of omega-3 – sourced in particular from oily fish – on reducing aggressive behaviour in both children and adults.[37]

'Deceptive tactics'

Although women and mothers often play pivotal roles in the purchase and preparation of children's food, they are not solely responsible for the food young people eat. In June 2024 the World Health Organization published a report into the way big industry fuels chronic diseases, obstructs health policy and targets vulnerable people. It called out just four corporate products as being responsible for 34 per cent of all deaths globally: tobacco, alcohol, fossil fuels, and ultra-processed food.[38] 'A small number of powerful transnational corporations wield significant power over the political and legal contexts in which they operate, and obstruct public interest regulations which could impact their profit margins,' the report said. Clearly the way that UPF companies, including those who manufacture formula milk and children's food, manipulate the food narrative, and even our own thoughts and desires, needs to be urgently addressed. The WHO describes this directly as 'deceptive tactics' from 'the industry playbook', and calls for action at the level of government and policy. But this does not mean that as individuals we can only wait helplessly for action. Just knowing that you are being manipulated makes it harder for you to be manipulated.

Since writing this book I've found myself really noticing product packaging, placement and advertising in a new way, and seeing it all with a much more cynical eye. When I look at a product like Pringles now, or Coca-Cola, and realize they are tempting me because of a lifetime of advertising and brand association and that, in reality, I probably won't enjoy them and definitely won't get any nutritional benefit from them, I find myself going off the idea. When I'm hungry and drive past a fast-food restaurant, instead of feeling tempted, I can think only of meat glue (see page 154). The selling points of take-out – that the food comes quickly and tastes just the same no matter where in the world you order it – now seem as unappealing to me as the pappy, spongy, bread-like substance each burger is served in. I think, if we are parents, or if we have kids in our life, we need to gently open their eyes in the same way. The best and healthiest way to do this is probably not by talking to them endlessly about how terrible UPF is, but rather to instil in them a curiosity and excitement about the colours, flavours and textures of food, and a love of cooking and eating. Allow them to chop veg and fruit in the kitchen, or stir the pot, or mix the crumble topping (they are rubbish at this and it ends up lumpy, by the way, but tastes roughly the same). Let them sniff a freshly sliced clove of garlic or a hunk of ginger. Keep food simple – repetitive even – it doesn't have to be complex, time-consuming or expensive: pasta with cheese and broccoli, or an egg, fried potato and carrots will do just fine. Make proper popcorn with them and watch it magically exploding with its mind-boggling twenty-five times volume expansion. Don't tell them that certain foods are 'not allowed' – just don't have them in the house, and steer away from them as much as possible, but not to the point of ruining birthday parties, where the entire spread will inevitably be UPF central. Make eating at a table together a priority – did you know that research has shown that teenagers consume UPF mindlessly and compulsively when they are in front of a screen?[39] And slowly but surely teach them to be critical thinkers, just as you perhaps do with the internet and social media, encouraging them to ask, 'what is the source?' and 'what is the motivation of the source?', when they are drawn to particular products. I write this with the 20/20 hindsight of someone who has made a lot of mistakes but who is hoping, as my youngest is still only ten years old, that it's not too late to turn things around. When we know better, we do better.

5.

Ben? Jerry? I'm breaking up with you!

Obesity and women's toxic relationship with UPF

In writing about body fat in the context of a book solely about women and food, it's important to be clear about a few things before we go further. First and foremost, if you are living with overweight or obesity, it is not your fault. In fact, this chapter will show quite the opposite – that the corporate greed of UPF manufacturers over the last few decades is squarely to blame. Like an abusive partner, they have manipulated all of us into believing they have our best interests at heart, whilst at the same time damaging us and making it very difficult for us to leave.

Secondly, the existing evidence, much of which controls for factors such as obesity, shows us that *all* people, regardless of their weight, are negatively affected by a diet high in UPF – so obese women are not being singled out in any way, nor am I going to suggest that anyone, of any size, needs to change that size unless they want to. Instead, this chapter is about exposing the toxic grip that UPF has on all women and, in doing so, offering a lifeline, a way out. Once you begin to realize that you are in a relationship where only one side is benefitting and the other is being callously put at risk, it may stop feeling like a good idea to keep investing in that relationship. Time's up: it's not you, it's UPF; this isn't good for you; you deserve better.

Women's relationship with their bodies, and with food itself, is deeply complicated, and any focus on ideas about what we 'should' or 'should not' be eating, or on the amount of fat our bodies are carrying, is loaded with what for many women is a lifetime of anxiety and stigma. This chapter is not about adding to that, but simply about exposing the truth about obesity, UPF and women's health, so that women who want to break up with UPF can solidify their reasons and then develop an exit strategy. Our shared stigma and anxiety about our female bodies plays its own part in the story, too, uniquely priming us to develop unhelpful or even addictive relationships with UPF, and making us crave more of the very substances that are causing us harm. Once we begin to see that the 'comfort' or 'treat' that UPF offers is part of a toxic cycle that relies on our emotional pain and low self-esteem, the idea of crying over a tub of ultra-processed ice cream might seem less appealing. We need to break free.

Obesity: the stats

Since the 1970s, the world's population has been getting bigger, with the number of people living with obesity globally surpassing one billion in 2022. The World Obesity Federation predicts that more than half of the global population will be overweight or obese by 2035.[1] In the UK, the Health Survey for England 2021 estimates that 25.9 per cent of adults in England are now obese and a further 37.9 per cent are overweight but not obese.[2] The Organisation for Economic Co-operation and Development (OECD) states that more than one in two adults and nearly one in six children are overweight or obese in much of Europe, Australasia, and North America.[3] And in the USA, figures show that between 1970 and 2020, obesity in adults increased by 20 per cent, and severe obesity by 10 per cent. The average American's BMI in 1971 was 25.7, today it is 30 – and this is the globally accepted threshold for obesity, meaning that the average American meets this threshold.

Overall, this is a trend that affects you regardless of your sex. In children and young people, obesity seems to be more prevalent among boys, with 50 million girls and 74 million boys worldwide living with obesity in 2019.[4] In adults, however, the figures vary depending on the country, with Western men tending more towards obesity than women, whilst globally the rates are higher for females, increasing from 69 million women in 1975 to 390 million in 2016, compared with 31 million men in 1975 increasing to 281 million in the same time period.[5] In women in the USA, severe obesity – defined as a BMI on or above 40 – has now reached nearly 12 per cent, almost double that of their male counterparts. Obesity is now considered an epidemic and, for the first time in human history, a greater risk to global public health than hunger.

Is UPF to blame?

As the number of people living with obesity has risen steadily, researchers and experts have sought explanations, and the most frequently offered over the past five decades have been:

- people are eating more;
- people are moving less;
- too much sugar;
- too much fat.

Untangling this is complicated, and probably constitutes a book in itself – in fact, there are dozens of existing books dedicated to these topics, many of which contradict each other. Yes, we probably are eating more; yes, we eat foods laden with sugar; yes, our lives are way more sedentary than they were less than a century ago, and all of these factors have an impact on our lives and health. But it seems like UPF is doing something *different* to our bodies, and that effect can't be explained simply by saying that UPF contains a lot of sugar, for example (which it does). Remember the Kevin Hall study (see page 40)? Hall gave people two different diets, one UPF and one non-UPF, that had *the exact same nutritional content*. Both diets contained roughly the same salt, sugar, fat and fibre. But on the UPF diet, participants not only ate around 500 calories more a day, they gained weight, about a kilogram, and they gained body fat, too.

Why? Research is ongoing, but there are a few likely answers. One is that the ultra-processing is changing the texture of the food, stripping it of fibre and making it unnaturally soft and much easier to eat, swallow and even digest quickly. This means we eat more of it than we ever could be bothered to do with whole food. Another related theory is that of 'hyperpalatability', a term coined by psychologist and addiction specialist Tera Fazzino, who describes how hyperpalatable foods (HPF), for example ready meals and salty snacks, are different from fresh or whole foods that occur in nature.[6] She explains:

> 'An apple, for example, typically has just one main palatability-related nutrient, the bit that makes it taste good, in this case sugar. This is combined with satiety-promoting nutrients, the ones that make us feel we have eaten enough, for example fibre, and water. But hyperpalatable foods are different. They have several different palatability-inducing nutrients, often combinations of fat, sugar and salt, at levels that simply don't occur in nature. Added to this, the nutrients that make us feel full, like the fibre, are often stripped away by the processing, making them readily absorbed into our system. So we may gain weight through HPF simply because they are tasty and difficult to stop eating.'

Fazzino's research has also found that the companies most likely to be responsible for creating and disseminating HPF into our food system knew a thing or two about creating addictive products designed for over-consumption – because they were very often owned by tobacco companies.[7] Her findings suggest that between 1988 and 2001, large numbers of major international food brands – from Kraft, to Birds Eye, to Lunchables – were owned by tobacco giants Philip Morris and R. J. Reynolds, and that their brands were as much as 80 per cent more likely to be HPF. Whilst tobacco companies divested from the US food system in the early 2000s, Fazzino believes that 'the shadow of big tobacco remained', as did many of the hyperpalatable products created during this time. This selective dissemination of HPF into the food system by companies whose very existence depended on the manipulation of human craving and the denial of any negative impact on public health is important to know not just for policy-makers tackling obesity, but for all of us as individuals when we reach for that second packet of crisps without really knowing why. Everything about UPF, even the marketing and packaging, is designed to make us eat more than we need.

Then there's the 'food matrix', which we met in Chapter 2 (see page 46), which refers to the molecular structure of the food that is often broken down by ultra-processing. We don't fully understand how this matrix interacts with the human body, but we do know that food that is broken down, for example fruit juice concentrate, has a very different effect on our blood sugar than, for example, whole fruit. Calorie-dense UPF may also lack nutrients that our bodies crave, causing us to feel hungry even after a meal, and there are also complex interactions between our taste buds – often over-stimulated by the complex flavours of UPF – and our guts, that may mean our bodies are primed in some way to expect nutrition they simply don't receive, messing with our metabolism and appetite. The gut microbiome (explored in detail in Chapter 6) – those huge numbers of bacteria that live in our digestive system – is also an area of importance here: we know that eating a diet high in UPF and low in plant- and fibre-rich foods (sometimes referred to as prebiotics) depletes the gut microbiome, and that people with obesity often have a very different and less diverse gut microbiome than those who are not obese. One 2023 study that focused specifically on women found a different gut bacterial make-up in those eating a diet high in UPF, and an association between this and leptin resistance.[8] Leptin is a hormone that helps with weight regulation; if you have leptin resistance, you are likely to feel hungry and driven to keep eating, even when your body already has enough fat stores.

And then there is the question of additives – are specific UPF ingredients interacting with our microbiome or another aspect of our biology and making us gain weight in ways that we are yet to fully understand? Researchers at the University of Paris have found that people eating a diet high in emulsifiers – commonly found in UPF – were more likely to develop Type 2 diabetes,[9] even when taking into account other risk factors, such as obesity and smoking, and the same research team found similar links between emulsifiers and cardiovascular disease.[10] One theory as to why this may be is that these emulsifiers disrupt the gut microbes, leading to inflammation, but there is clearly much that we don't yet know.

Some important points to note

- There is a link between a diet high in UPF and being overweight or obese – this is now supported by numerous studies.
- Stopping or reducing UPF won't necessarily lead to weight loss if you are eating more food than you need. Overweight people existed before the advent of UPF.
- Stopping or reducing UPF and instead eating a balanced diet with ingredients from Nova 1, 2 and 3 cannot *harm* your health in any way. Organizations or experts that suggest that UPF categories are 'too confusing' or that there may be a risk to cutting back on UPF are almost always linked to Big Food companies.
- The health issues associated with UPF affect people of every size. Cutting down or quitting UPF is good for everybody's health.

In fact, it's potentially hard to separate out the harms to your health brought about by high BMI from those brought about by a diet high in UPF. We know that, for all people living with obesity, there are increased risks of many of the major diseases, such as heart disease, stroke, diabetes and cancer.[11] We also know that eating UPF increases the risk of these diseases in people who are not obese. No person – male, female, obese, not obese – benefits from a diet high in UPF.

The specific impact of obesity on women's health

In women, being obese is associated with a range of female-specific health issues, for example lowered fertility.[12] Women living with obesity often have irregular menstrual cycles and ovulate less, making both natural conception and in vitro fertilization (IVF) treatment more difficult. Pregnancy complications like gestational diabetes and pre-eclampsia are more common in obese women, as is gestational hypertension (high blood pressure in the second half of pregnancy), sleep apnea (when you temporarily stop breathing during your sleep), and a higher chance of miscarriage. Obesity also brings increased symptoms of polycystic ovary syndrome (PCOS), a hormonal condition that can cause irregular periods, fertility issues, facial hair growth and acne.

Female cancers, like breast, womb and ovarian cancer, are all higher in obese women, with the risk increasing the more weight is gained and the longer it is held for.[13] Obesity causes cancer because the fat in our body, rather than being passive and inactive as you might imagine, is actually sending out signals to the body, releasing hormones and communicating with other organs. For example, immune cells go to areas of the body where there are a lot of fat cells, which causes inflammation, which in turn can cause cells to divide quicker, potentially increasing cancer risk. In the case of breast cancer, there is a strong obesity link: about 9 per cent of women of a healthy weight will develop breast cancer after fifty years of age, but in those living with obesity this figure is more like 12 per cent.[14] This is because women who are obese will continue to produce oestrogen at higher levels, even in menopause, and this can make cells in the breast divide, increasing the likelihood of cancer. Excess oestrogen caused by obesity raises the risk of womb cancer, too.

It's important to stress again that the risk of eating UPF applies to everyone: in the case of ovarian cancer, for example, researchers in 2023 used the Nova classification to look at the impact of UPF on cancer rates. They followed a huge cohort of nearly 200,000 people and found that, even when adjusting for other risk factors, like smoking, high BMI and sociodemographics, every 10 per cent increase in UPF consumption was associated with a 6 per cent increase of dying from cancer of any kind – but this risk was noticeably higher for women's cancers. The researchers found that, with each additional 10 per cent increase in UPF consumption, there was a 16 per cent increase in the risk of dying from breast cancer and a 30 per cent increased risk of dying from ovarian cancer.[15]

UPF is damaging to all women's health. It is also making some women obese and this obesity is causing further health damage and complications. The debilitating and painful condition endometriosis, which affects one in ten women, is more likely to be found in women with a BMI in the 'healthy' range, but those women with endometriosis and obesity have been found to score twice as high on severity of symptoms.[16] Menopause is made worse by obesity: studies have found that women with a high BMI have worse symptoms, like 'hot flashes',[17] and that they may find HRT less effective.[18] Alzheimer's disease, which affects twice as many women as men, and other forms of dementia are all made more likely by obesity – with several studies demonstrating that those who are obese in mid-life may have their dementia risk increased by as much as 30 per cent.

Obesity also affects women's mental health, and disproportionately so, perhaps because of the cultural pressure that so many women feel to be thin and the stigma perpetuated about larger female bodies. The relationship between obesity and depression, for example, is significantly higher in women.[19] Obesity and depression are inextricably linked in that depression increases the risk for obesity and obesity increases the risk for depression, but one study has found depressed obese women have higher leptin levels,[20] which we know is also associated with high UPF consumption.[21] With low self-esteem, too, obesity both drives this and is driven by it in turn, although events such as sudden bereavement, which have been shown to impact self-esteem, can also trigger weight gain due to increased eating and decreased activity, particularly in females.[22] Obese women who have tried to lose weight but been unable to do so are significantly more likely to think about suicide; the same is not true of obese males.[23] Living with obesity can affect women's quality of life, body image, and sex lives. Obesity is associated with an impaired ability to orgasm in women[24] and with lack of enjoyment of sexual activity, lack of sexual desire, difficulties with sexual performance, and avoidance of sexual encounters.[25] Again, all of these associations are far more prevalent in women than they are in men.

One apple is enough

It seems like there's an obvious answer for anyone living with overweight or obesity, or who simply wants to make a change: stop eating UPF. But that's complicated and hard for a number of reasons. For some, it's about time and convenience; others may lack the know-how or have concerns about cost. Going forwards, there's a role for governments and policy-makers to play in making food that is not ultra-processed more accessible, and perhaps upskilling a generation of people in ways of being less reliant on these products. But it's also interesting to think about the reasons why women have become overweight in the first place, and why they often find it incredibly difficult or impossible to return to a healthy weight. We know that obesity has a genetic component, but that doesn't explain the rising rates over the past five decades. And we know that UPF is hyperpalatable, making us want the whole packet of biscuits in a way that we would rarely experience with an apple – one apple is almost always enough. But let's think about the person eating the packet of biscuits for a moment (perhaps it's you), and remember that their reasons for doing so might be very different depending on whether they are male or female.

Women's eating patterns and motivations are different from men's. First, our brains are different, specifically in areas connected to appetite regulation and energy maintenance. Researchers at UCLA, for example, looked at male and female brains and found that the drivers for overeating were different according to sex.[26] Women who were obese showed more prominent changes in the brain's reward system related to dopamine responsiveness, suggesting that emotion-related eating and compulsive eating play a larger role for them, whereas obese men's brains showed more signs of remodelling in sensorimotor regions, a sign that their eating behaviour is more affected by gut sensations and physical discomfort. Numerous other studies have reached similar conclusions: women are more likely than men to turn to food for comfort when stressed, angry, depressed, anxious or upset.[27] We don't fully understand why this is – it could be to do with gendered expectations around emotions, or perhaps a means of self-medication. What we do know is that the food women turn to is very likely to be UPF: chocolate, biscuits, crisps, pizza, ice cream. I mean, when was the last time you stress-ate a banana?

Scientists think the reason for this is the unique make-up of UPF that you don't find in any other type of food and the 'high' it delivers, specifically the ratio of carbs to fat.[28] That apple that you only want one of – it's got a carbs to fat ratio of 36:1. A piece of salmon has a carbs to fat ratio of 0:1. But an industrially made chocolate bar? That has the magic and very unnatural ratio that simply doesn't occur in nature: 1:1. In other words, it has carbs and fat in equal measure. Not only this, but the *levels* of carbs and fat in the chocolate bar are way higher than you would find in nature, too.

100 g	Carbohydrate	Fat	Ratio
Apple	55 kcal	1.5 kcal	36:1
Salmon	0 kcal	73 kcal	0:1
Chocolate	237 kcal	266 kcal	1:1

So UPF is a substance our human bodies have only experienced in the past few decades of our history – and it delivers an unmatchable hit. Boom! Carbs and fat, incoming, and fast. There are some foods in nature that are higher in carbs and fat than apples or salmon, for example almonds (86 kcal of carbs and 449 kcal of fat, giving them a 1:5 ratio), but have you ever tried to eat them fast? (Don't.) They have that pesky food matrix that means you have to chew them up in a painstakingly slow way compared to your Cadbury's Flake, and when they do finally hit your stomach, they take much longer to digest. There's simply not the same instant high that we women may seek when we feel low.

In this way you could argue that women are uniquely primed to be victims of the UPF industry, particularly when you consider UPF is now thought by some to be an addictive substance, and even more so when you take into account that UPF has been found to play a big role in eating disorders, particularly binge-eating disorder, where a person is regularly compelled to eat more than they need over a short space of time. These 'hyperpalatable' foods that deliver their fast, intense and unique hit are causing a unique new kind of addiction, 'ultra-processed food addiction', and a unique new kind of eating disorder, 'ultra-processed food use disorder', say psychologists. Reaching for the UPF when you are unhappy or emotional has a powerful effect on the brain's reward system, in similar ways to smoking or substance abuse. Our brains are then primed to seek out another similar hit, firing up the dopamine cravings when we so much as see the packaging or the golden arches. This explains why we find ourselves adding crisps and chocolate to the trolley or heading into KFC even when we know it's 'bad for us'. Added to this, the more high-fat-high-carbs food we eat, the less interested our brain becomes in the low-fat options.[29] Like an abusive partner cutting us off from friends, family and the activities we love, UPF ensures our options are narrowed so that we only have them to turn to. Nothing else can make us feel as good as UPF does.

Ultra-processed food disorder is as yet not an official diagnosis, but there have already been observations of the role of UPF in existing eating disorders, all of which are far more prevalent in women and girls. Those with eating disorders that involve binging, such as bulimia and binge-eating disorder, are likely to use 100 per cent UPF during binging episodes,[30] and have also been found to have diets high in UPF – as high as 70 per cent.[31] These two types of eating disorder have also been consistently shown to have strong associations with childhood trauma and abuse, which we know is far more prevalent in girls, in particular sexual abuse, which is over three times more likely to happen to females.[32] And girls who have experienced childhood sexual abuse are more than twice as likely to go on to develop binge-eating disorder, and nearly three times as likely to develop bulimia.[33] Whilst women and girls with eating disorders are not always obese, child abuse has been found to be a predictor of adult obesity, with victims citing the desire to 'desexualise' their bodies, make themselves more 'physically imposing', be less 'noticeable' or build a 'protective wall'.[34] UPF presents itself as 'comfort' for our emotional distress, but in fact it is just another abuser in disguise.

'Stop dieting, start losing weight' (SlimFast slogan, 2003)

Many women, regardless of their weight, dislike what they see when they look in the mirror, particularly when naked. In *The Beauty Myth*, Naomi Wolf describes the 'One Stone Solution', a phenomenon in which women who are not overweight feel that they need to lose fourteen pounds in order to become their ideal selves. The attempt to lose this stone leads to an endless cycle of dieting and weight gain from which we can never escape, and Wolf does not see it as a coincidence that this reinforcement of women as failures began in the decades during which we were beginning to have a more equal share of success. Dieting keeps us focused on ourselves and our reflection in the mirror, it is 'the most potent political sedative in women's history', she writes. *The Beauty Myth* was published in 1990, when obesity rates were only fifteen years into their meteoric rise, and when the 'diet industry' was only just getting off the blocks. Now, not only do we have much larger numbers of women living with obesity, we also have increasingly extreme 'solutions', from surgery to weight-loss injections. Whilst obesity affects both men and women, nearly 80 per cent of bariatric surgery is carried out on females,[35] and women are substantially more likely to want to try drugs like Ozempic and Wegovy than men[36] – perhaps because weight loss and the search for the perfect body is still a predominantly female preoccupation. UPF companies are said to be concerned about the advent of these drugs, which suppress appetite and slow digestion, with Nestlé reportedly hinting in October 2023 that it is already working on products 'specifically intended to meet consumers' appetite suppressed needs'.[37] They may not need to worry – the weight-loss drugs are costly and need to be taken on an ongoing basis. If stopped, and UPF consumption rises again, the weight loss will be reversed.

In every supermarket you will find several kinds of UPF that make claims about weight loss. From the most obvious products, like SlimFast shakes, to the more ubiquitous, such as 'calorie controlled' ready meals, 'slimline' or 'diet' sodas, '90 calorie chocolate brownies', 'Go Ahead Fruit & Oat Bakes' and the 'low calorie' ice cream that plays on decades of messaging about 'good' and 'sinful' foods by calling itself 'Halo', the shelves are weighed down with UPFs that come with a side order of self-improvement. All of them ultra-processed, all of them manufactured by the same factories, companies and using many of the same UPF ingredients that are driving mindless eating, food addiction and obesity. Similar to the tobacco companies that created products like 'low tar' cigarettes and now vapes, simply to appear more 'healthy' whilst continuing to make profit, a 'sin free' cake is not going to help you to lose weight any more than Marlboro Lights are going to reduce your risk of cancer. Quite the contrary, you will still be eating UPF and simultaneously reinforcing your own expectations of certain tastes and textures and types of food at certain times of day. You will be staying in the toxic relationship. You could have an apple, of course, but that might put Mr Kipling out of a job. And it probably goes without saying that Mr Kipling's unlikely to be found eating a 'FitBake': these 'diet' products are almost overwhelmingly marketed at women.

Whilst smoking is different from eating in that everyone has to eat to stay alive, there are many parallels between the tactics of UPF companies and those used historically by the makers of cigarettes and tobacco. Like the tobacco companies, food companies also seek 'health by association' messaging – just as Virginia Slims sponsored women's tennis, Coca-Cola sponsors the Olympics. Money flows from both industries into 'good causes', often related to the same groups that are targeted and damaged by their products – people from lower socio-economic backgrounds, women, children. McVitie's has partnered with a mental health charity; McDonald's has long run Ronald McDonald's House for children; many make extended claims about their support for the environment. Rather like the doctors who endorsed smoking, messaging about UPF comes from organizations that sound like they have our best interests at heart: the British Nutrition Foundation, for example, tells us in its position statement about UPF that, 'blanket advice to avoid ultra-processed foods may have unintended consequences that have not been fully investigated for different groups within the population'.[38] But the British Nutrition Foundation has corporate members that include British Sugar, Coca-Cola, Greggs PLC and Mars UK Ltd.[39]

Like the tobacco industry, the food industry also courts friends in high places – in the UK, the government has been 'assailed by lobbyists' opposed to proposed restrictions on food advertising and meal deals,[40] MPs have been given free giant bars of Dairy Milk, and KFC has been accused of pressuring councils over child obesity policies, such as a veto on branches of their restaurant being opened near schools.[41] In the USA, Kraft Heinz has 'improved' the nutritional content of its 'Lunchables' – a plastic pack of crackers, reformed ham, processed cheese and an Oreo – so they can be part of the National School Lunch Program.⁴² In the meantime their CEO, Carlos Abrams-Rivera, has told the *Wall Street Journal* that he's a fan of clean eating, intermittent fasting and follows a mostly Mediterranean diet.⁴³ Like the tobacco companies – yes, the same ones that used to be the parent company to Kraft Heinz, which produces Lunchables – the CEOs of Big Food almost certainly think of such anomalies as a matter of freedom and personal choice. When their heads hit their luxury pillows after a nice grilled chicken salad, they presumably sleep well, believing that they are freely making 'good' choices, while others freely make 'bad' ones.

Breaking free

This messaging, that 'all food is good for you' and 'you just have to make the right choices', is at odds with the public health crisis of obesity. It's also quite deliberate, placing all of the emphasis for change on the individual, and letting the food companies off the hook. The exact same tactic was used by tobacco companies again and again in the second half of the twentieth century to prevent legislation against cigarette-smoking. By framing smoking as an issue of freedom, that people didn't have to do if they didn't want to, it made any argument against smoking seem like a really mean, killjoy attack on free choices. But smoking was heavily advertised and promoted, highly addictive, and also often marketed towards the young (for example, by the cartoon 'Joey the Camel' on Camel cigarettes), hooking them in early, in spite of the overwhelming evidence of the risks to health. With UPF, there's a very similar pattern – a narrative that suggests people can take or leave UPF, and that all the food companies are doing is providing us with options. Often, as with tobacco, it's people from poorer socio-economic backgrounds who are both targeted by the marketing and face the greatest damage to health. Rather than offering freedom, UPF imprisons many in repetitive and inescapable cycles.

I realize that breaking any toxic cycle – addiction, destructive relationships – is complex and multi-factorial. But certainly a good step is the moment the scales fall from our eyes and we realize: I am not benefitting in any way from this; this is not love. What is being promised here is not actually being delivered, and I am being manipulated and damaged by someone or something that really doesn't give a stuff about me. And once we've had this revelation, the rest is just a matter of extricating ourselves. In real terms this means that when we hook up with that frozen pizza or packet of ready-made cakes, we see it in a new light. No longer do we believe the lies that this 'food' is fun, a treat, a convenience, a choice. In fact, it's not really 'food' at all, but an unnatural and habit-forming substance that is liable to make us eat much more than we need, and may be altering our bodies in ways we still don't really understand. It may well make us gain an unhealthy amount of weight, which will bring us a unique set of health issues, but even if it doesn't, it's likely to bring us a few health issues anyway. Ending it may take time and willpower, but sorry UPF, the love has gone. It's over.

6.

An apple a day keeps the OBGYN away

The care and feeding of your female microbiome

I can still remember the moment when I first heard that bacteria weren't just little gremlins you needed to bleach off your toilet. It was the summer of 2013 and, pregnant with my third child, I was in the midst of moving from our rented cottage to a dilapidated renovation project. I had a two-year-old and a five-year-old at the time, who were, frankly, not a great deal of help with the whole packing thing, and I was also writing a popular weekly column about all things birth and parenting for the UK magazine *Best*. Seven months pregnant and sat on the floor surrounded by boxes that had been packed by me and then unpacked again by toddlers, I was speaking to Toni Harman about a piece I was working on. Toni had directed the 2012 documentary film *Freedom for Birth*, a film about the persecuted home-birth midwife Ágnes Geréb and the wider picture of women's rights and autonomy in childbirth globally. I can't remember what I was picking Toni's brains about that day, but just as we were saying goodbye at the end of the conversation, I asked her what she was working on next, and she said,

'Have you heard of the human microbiome? We're working on a film about that.'

I had absolutely nothing in the file under the word 'microbiome'. I don't think many people did in the early 2010s. I listened patiently as Toni explained enthusiastically about what she said was going to be THE topic everyone would soon be talking about. She told me the basics, that we all had these colonies of bacteria that live on our skin, and in our guts, and that scientists were discovering that they could have a huge impact on our health. It was also thought that the way a baby was born – either vaginally or via caesarean – could affect the microbes that person had in their own personal colony, maybe even for life. 'This is going to be the next big thing, Milli, it's going to change everything, it's like the discovery of a whole new universe!,' said Toni. I respected her greatly but – maybe it was the stress of our impending move to a building site with two, soon to be three, small humans in tow – I have to be honest and say I thought she had completely lost the plot. It just sounded too far-fetched. I said my goodbyes and promptly forgot the topic.

But Toni had not lost the plot – in fact, she'd been incredibly prescient. Since we spoke that day in 2013, knowledge and understanding of our resident bacteria has snowballed – or should I say, mushroomed. It's become a buzz topic, with most people at least vaguely aware of concepts like 'gut health', and even celebrities like Paris Hilton getting on board with companies offering at-home tests, whereby you can send off your poop and get a full report on exactly what's living in your intestines. Although there's a lot of focus on gut bacteria, we now know that there are other colonies all over our bodies – on our skin, up our noses and in our respiratory tract, in our mouths, in our urinary system, in our eyes, in our lungs, and, if we are female, in our vagina and reproductive tract.

There is also emerging research to suggest there are microbiomes in other areas, for example the brain, the uterus, and even the placenta, but this is still being studied. Each area known to have microbes has its own distinctive balance of species and, to a certain extent, these differ from person to person. However, it would be simplistic to think of each microbiome – gut, skin, vagina, etc. – as separate. Rather than working in isolation, they are all parts of a whole and have relationships with each other or with organs of the body, sometimes referred to as their 'axis', for example the gut-brain axis. It's a vast, interconnected ecosystem, and the interactions between we humans and our various resident colonies, and between the colonies themselves, are numerous and complex, as are their roles in our health and disease.

Scientists are also delving into new understandings of sex differences in the microbiome – yes, male and female microbiomes seem to be different. Some refer to this study of sex differences in our bacterial colonies as the 'microgenderome', whilst others argue that since gender is a social construct and tends to relate to ideas about masculinity and femininity, we should talk about the 'microsexome', because the factors that drive its binary male or female differences are determined by biological sex, not by gender.[1] Whether you choose to say microgenderome or microsexome, the fascinating reality is that there seem to be differences in the male and female microbiomes even before puberty, at which point they intensify.[2] As our knowledge of the microsexome develops, it potentially holds the key to sex-based health disparities, for example the greater prevalence in women of gut issues like irritable bowel syndrome (IBS), or auto-immune disorders such as Lupus and Multiple sclerosis (MS).[3] In our lifetimes, greater understanding of the role of the microsexome in health may transform such women's lives.

In a field that currently has many more questions than answers, the bacterial colonies that inhabit areas of the body that are unique to women are perhaps the least understood. This, say researchers, is due to the disproportionate allocation of funding towards disorders more prevalent in males, leaving us with a 'significant knowledge gap'.[4] The studies we do have are also not racially representative, all of which means that most of our information set is likely to be based on the microbes of white Western industrialized men. The microbiome, comprised of microorganisms including fungi, protozoa, archaea, viruses and microbiota, is estimated to be as much as ten times greater than the total number of cells in the human body, and it's thought that their genetic information is at least 150 times greater than that of the human genome.[5] But its overall diversity is low when compared with non-industrialized humans, in particular hunter-gatherer populations, who have extremely diverse microbiomes. Our Western microbial depletion is thought to be due to several factors: antibiotic use, caesarean birth and formula milk, highly sanitized living environments, loss of contact with animals and the soil, and the consumption of highly processed foods.[6]

Why might UPF be impacting on all of our microbiomes, whether we are male or female? In part, this will be due to the wholefoods that are being displaced when we fill ourselves up with UPF – it's about what we are *not* eating. It's widely accepted that the microbiome thrives when we eat 'non-digestible carbohydrates from plants' – in other words, fibre. These cell walls of plants, sometimes referred to as 'prebiotics', are fermented by the gut bacteria and produce short chain fatty acids, which have all kinds of brilliant health benefits. But UPF is notoriously low in fibre and does not contain these plant cell walls (you'll recall how intense processing breaks down the structure or the 'matrix' of food). As well as the benefits we miss for our microbiome when we eat UPF rather than plants, there are also studies that suggest typical UPF additives, such as emulsifiers,[7] sweeteners,[8] maltodextrin[9] and xanthan gum,[10] could be at best altering, and at worst harming, our microbiome.[11]

You are what you eat

Less than a year after Toni Harman had boggled my mind with the very first thoughts I'd ever had about this new frontier, my editor at *Best* asked me to write a piece about 'new birth trends', including one that I was suddenly hearing a lot of talk about amongst those working in maternity services. The practice, known as 'seeding the microbiome' or 'microbirthing' (in part after the film Toni went on to make: *Microbirth*), seemed to draw a collective gasp of shock when the article went live. Women who were due to give birth via planned caesarean section were placing a piece of gauze in their vagina prior to surgery, and then wiping this gauze on the baby after birth, in order to mimic the way that bacteria would 'colonize' the baby if it were born vaginally. Some women were doing this off their own bat and without 'permission' (not that you need it, it's your baby and your vagina), whilst others were being encouraged and supported by doctors or midwives. All involved believed that this 'seeding' could potentially mitigate some of the increased future health risks that studies show are associated with being born by caesarean, for example of obesity, asthma, eczema, and Type 2 diabetes.

How we come to review this practice twenty, thirty or three hundred years down the track remains to be seen. Already it seems to be a fading trend, with both concerns about the possibility of infection from the wrong kind of bacteria, like Group B strep, and also with growing understanding about other ways to influence the microbiome, for example through breastfeeding and, later in life, diet. The women who, rightly or wrongly, seeded their babies in the 2010s were responding to two key pieces of information: first, that the microbiome of newborn babies was different, depending on the mode of delivery; and second, that by 'microbirthing', the microbiome of a caesarean-born baby could be made more similar – but not identical – to that of a baby born vaginally. People were immediately divided by these new ideas. Perhaps, just like me when I first spoke to Toni, it was simply too much for them to initially compute. And, as well as being a completely alien, brand-new and complex field of emerging science, added into the mix was the somewhat upsetting idea that one type of birth might be 'better' for a baby's health than another. Also, perhaps worse still, was all the talk of vaginal fluids and of rubbing them on a newborn baby's face, which some people seemed to find a bit 'icky' – as if vaginas and newborn babies were not usually seen in the same room.

Rather than being icky, vaginal fluids are a bit special. The vagina has its own unique microbiome: a little colony of mostly one genus of bacteria, called lactobacillus. In the gut microbiome you're aiming for diversity – a healthy gut microbiome is thought to be one with as many species as possible, a bit like a rich and thriving rainforest. With the vagina, the opposite is best: you are aiming for simplicity. Just a handful of different types of lactobacillus, whose role is to produce lactic acid, serving as a protective barrier against pathogens and maintaining a balanced 'ecosystem'. Ina Schuppe Koistinen, an associate professor at the Karolinska Institutet in Sweden, is an expert in the vaginal microbiome, and gives this advice: 'Maintaining a healthy vaginal microbiome is simpler than it seems – avoid soaps and douches, opt for breathable cotton underwear, and focus on a balanced diet rich in probiotics and fibre. Using condoms with new sexual partners is also important, as it helps protect the delicate microbial balance. These small, everyday habits can go a long way in supporting your vaginal health naturally.'

If I asked you how you could upset the balance of your own vaginal ecosystem, you might come up with some ideas: fragranced soaps, perfumes, or maybe even antibiotics. But what's absolutely crucial, and perhaps less obvious, is that this vital little colony is influenced by what you eat. Not only this, but the difference between a healthy and 'dysbiotic' vagina could potentially have a huge impact on multiple areas of women's health.

Happy gut = happy vagina

Ever heard of the oestrobolome? No, I hadn't either. It's the name for the collection of bacteria in our gut that is capable of metabolizing and modulating oestrogen. Men have an oestrobolome in their gut, too (and if you're in the USA, it's the estrobolome). For some reason, I picture the oestrobolome looking a bit like Ursula the Sea Witch from Disney's *The Little Mermaid*, and although there is nothing villainous about it, I suppose it does have great power and influence on what happens up nearer the surface of our bodies, and our minds, too, from way down in the dark, murky depths.

An oestrobolome that's functioning optimally, and maintaining optimal oestrogen levels, is incredibly important for women's health. The oestrobolome functions best, metabolizing and eliminating just the right amounts of oestrogen, with the help of a diverse gut microbiome, and the key to this is a diet that's rich in vegetables, fruit, whole grains, nuts, seeds, berries, herbs, beans and pulses – all the stuff you get less of if you're eating a lot of UPF. It particularly likes fermenting those fibrous plant cell walls – so an apple a day really may keep the OBGYN away. If your oestrogen levels are too high, you can experience a range of issues, from endometriosis to cancer; if your oestrogen levels are too low, the colony of lactobacillus in your vagina will become depleted, making you vulnerable to infection.[12]

The vaginal microbiome differs from woman to woman, influenced by sexual activity, washing habits, stress, geographical location, race, and diet. The delicate balance of each woman's vaginal ecosystem, and its resident population of lactobacillus, is not fixed either, even when healthy – it changes with age, during pregnancy, and with the menstrual cycle. Before puberty, and after menopause, for example, the population of lactobacillus decreases, but if you take HRT it is restored to pre-menopausal levels. These fluctuations are because the lactobacillus 'feed' off something called glycogen, and glycogen goes up when levels of oestrogen are higher, and down when they are lower – it's all under the control of the Sea Witch, basically.

If you've ever had thrush, known officially as vulvovaginal candidiasis, you might have something in the file under 'Diet Vagina Connection'. There are a raft of books and websites on changing what you eat to try to get rid of persistent yeast infections by reducing overgrowth of candida albicans, which is actually not a bacteria but a fungi, and part of the mycobiome – the name for your resident sub-colony of fungi. Thrush can make life a misery, with persistent and recurring vaginal itching, discharge and soreness, and claims that a diet high in wholefoods and low in sugar will help are largely sneered at – you're more likely to be prescribed anti-fungal tablets or cream. But dietary changes, in particular increasing your intake of plant fibre for your gut bacteria to ferment, can up the lactobacilli in your vaginal microbiome and these have been shown – in a petri dish, at least – to reduce the growth of candida.

If you're one of the 20–30 per cent of women who suffer from bacterial vaginosis (BV), you'll also know the impact of a vaginal microbiome whose lactobacillus are all out of whack. Symptoms can include itching, pain, a fishy-smelling discharge, and a burning sensation when you pee – it's not pleasant. And it's not particularly brilliantly understood either. If you have symptoms, you're likely to get the same treatment women have been given for the past fifty years – oral or topical antibiotics – and in around 80 per cent of cases, it will come back. If you've noticed your symptoms fluctuating, perhaps with your menstrual cycle, this is almost certainly connected to the oestrobolome, and the shifting levels of oestrogen providing more or less glycogen to keep your lactobacillus colony happy. If the colony is depleted, bingo, your vagina's defences are lowered, and the resulting BV can have serious ramifications, including sexually transmitted infections, pelvic inflammatory disease, and even pregnancy complications, such as waters breaking early (PROM), preterm birth, and low birth weight.[13] And whilst anecdotally women with BV report rarely being asked about their diet, it's almost certainly a factor worth exploring: one 2022 study found that an 'unhealthy diet', high in sugar and fat and low in fruits and vegetables, raised the risk of BV.[14]

A happy vaginal microbiome with its well-balanced lactobacillus community may also reduce the risk of HPV infection (Human Papillomavirus) that is recognized to cause cervical cancer. Vaginas with higher numbers of certain strains of lactobacillus have been shown to clear HPV more efficiently, whereas vaginas with low lactobacillus and with some of the strains associated with BV have higher rates of HPV infection and persistence. This same vulnerability caused by low lactobacillus may well extend to other viruses, for example HIV, the virus that can progress to AIDS.[15] And the health of the vaginal microbiome is also directly related to issues such as Urinary Tract Infection (UTI), because the initial step for the infecting bacteria is to colonize the entrance to the vagina.[16] If the vagina is high in those fabulous lactobacilli, then their low pH will zap the pathogens before they even get going on their unpleasant plans for your urethra, bladder and kidneys.

The fact that there's a connection between bacterial infections and bacterial colonies may make some intuitive sense, but interestingly there are also emerging links between gut and vaginal bacteria and other women's health issues that may not seem quite so obvious, such as PCOS, uterine fibroids (UF), endometrial cancer and endometriosis. In Chapter 5, we touched on endometriosis, a debilitating condition in which cells similar to those from the lining of the womb grow in other places, such as the ovaries or fallopian tubes, causing chronic pain and, in some cases, fertility issues. Around one in ten women suffer with endometriosis, often waiting years for a diagnosis, and there is as yet no cure. Researchers have found differences in the gut, vaginal and endometrial microbiomes of women with endometriosis, and a number of studies have shown that diet could improve the condition.[17] These studies have recommended eating less red meat and trans fat (the latter is banned in the USA but still found in UK products such as UPF pastries, cakes and biscuits under names like 'hydrogenated fat', 'partially hydrogenated oils' and 'mono and diglycerides of fatty acids'), and more plant-based fibre – yes, just to repeat, this improves the diversity of our gut microbes and helps keep our oestrogen levels regulated. Similarly, researchers investigating PCOS and endometrial cancer have found changes in the microbiome, and in the case of fibroids have shown that increased intake of vitamin D slows their growth because of its improvement of gut microbe diversity. Future treatments for all these conditions, they say, will almost certainly involve manipulation of the microbiome – but in the meantime, you are of course able to manipulate it yourself, by replacing the UPF in your diet with wholefoods and plants.

Trust your gut

The idea that there is a 'gut-brain axis' is quite widely evidenced now – a complex network of communication between our gut and our brain in which the nervous system, the immune system, hormones and the microbiome are all thought to play a part. It seems like the bacteria in our intestines have a hotline to our brains (and the brain talks back), influencing not only our sense of intuition and 'gut reactions' but also, perhaps, our darkest emotions. In the UK and USA, women are twice as likely overall to experience depression as men, and twice as likely to have anxiety. Not only are there differences between the gut microbiomes of mentally and physically healthy males and females, but research has also shown changes in the gut microbiomes of women with depression and anxiety.

For me, having worked for several years as a therapist in my twenties, this potentially explains one of my greatest unanswered questions from that experience: what creates resilience? Why are some people able to come through adverse childhoods or traumatic experiences and have happy, successful lives, whilst others are less able to cope, and still others have a lifetime of struggling with devastating impacts of poor mental health? One of my jobs in the mid-2000s was in the NHS, working with a group of women with a diagnosis of borderline personality disorder (BPD) as part of a team of therapists with different approaches. Around 75 per cent of people diagnosed with BPD are female. All of the women in my group had experienced severe trauma as children or adults, often both; all of them had extremely painful and difficult emotional lives, struggling to regulate, cope, maintain relationships, or even feel anything at all. Many self-harmed or contemplated suicide regularly. But not all people who have such histories go on to find life difficult in this way. These women realized this, and often it only compounded their distress, as if their inability to cope made them lesser humans and this weakness of character had perhaps even made them easier victims in their abuse. None of this could possibly be true, of course, but it was often part of the intensely dark way they perceived themselves. Their disorder also meant that they were often extremely angry with me and anyone else on the team, but at the same time they were desperate to be helped. In all our therapeutic interventions, which were creative and wide-ranging, we never considered diet. Overall, I would say that the work we did with this group of women was of very little use to them – they left the programme as they had arrived, in deep, chronic distress. Only one study appears to have been done into the gut microbes of women with BPD, and the researchers found that four bacterial species were significantly less abundant.[18] Much more research is needed before we may potentially have an answer to the question that many women with BPD and other complex mental health issues often have: 'why me?'

More widely, we could also ask, 'why women?' Some of the answer, at least, seems to lie in the role oestrogen plays in the gut-brain axis – yes, it's the Sea Witch again. Some studies seem to hint that oestrogen, and progesterone too, along with the sex differences in the female microbiome may make the gut-brain axis in women unique and play a role in female mental health. But much of the research on the gut-brain axis to date has been exclusively focused on males, with not just women but even female mice being left out of the studies completely. The role that the fluctuating hormones of the menstrual cycle and the female life phases of pregnancy, perimenopause and post-menopause play in the microbiome's impact on our brains and emotions simply hasn't been researched.[19]

Not much is yet known either about whether UPF may have a different impact on the male and female microbiomes. One study in Spain looked specifically at how UPF might affect the microbiomes of men and women differently, and discovered that a diet high in UPF was associated with different strains of gut bacteria in women than in men. The most interesting finding of this study, in my opinion, was that the women on high UPF diets were five times more likely to suffer depression and three times more likely to suffer anxiety than men on the same high levels of UPF. There is so much more research to be done, but...imagine if the large and rising numbers of women with anxiety and depressive disorders could all be traced back to tiny microbes in the female gut?

Eating for two

Diet in pregnancy can feel like an area where women are patronized and policed, causing us yet more anxiety and guilt. Nevertheless, our growing understanding of the 'maternal microbiome' suggests that what we eat during pregnancy and breastfeeding is one of several factors that shape not only our own microbial health but that of our baby, too.[20] This is bad news in the sense that it potentially gives pregnant women something else to worry about, but good news in the sense that this emerging science is at least a bit more interesting than being told to go steady on the pâté.

During my own pregnancies, I ate with even more abandon than usual, feeling that 'all food was good food'. I was told that I 'didn't need to eat for two' by a few killjoys, but I largely chose to ignore them, seeing pregnancy as an opportunity to over-indulge without having to worry about my waistline for once. The alcohol, blue cheese, runny egg and rare steak guidelines irritated me, but apart from grumpily sticking to the rules and wondering why the French apparently find them ridiculous, I ate what I wanted and what I craved, without making much distinction between a pack of Doritos with supermarket dips and a lentil traybake. If I fancied it, I ate it.

Now it seems I could have been slightly more mindful. One of the least understood microbiomes is that of the uterus, the 'endometrial microbiome', but scientists are investigating its impact on both natural fertility and the effectiveness of fertility treatments.[21] Once pregnant, the maternal microbiome – of gut, endometrium, vagina and even the mouth – is influenced by diet as well as genetics, antibiotic use, infection and stress. Mouth bacteria, for example those that cause gum disease, have been shown to be associated with miscarriage,[22] low birth weight, and pre-eclampsia.[23] There is a growing body of evidence to suggest that the maternal microbiome plays a role in many adverse pregnancy outcomes (APOs), such as miscarriage, recurrent loss,[24] rupture of membranes before the end of pregnancy (PROM), hyperemesis gravidarum (commonly known as severe morning sickness), premature birth, growth restriction, and stillbirth. On paper, they are 'APOs', but in reality, each is a challenging and often devastating human story. Our understanding of the microbiome may offer us a future in which they do not wreak such damage.

As we will see in Chapter 7, UPF consumption in pregnancy has been linked to a range of health issues and poor outcomes, although in many cases this has not yet been proven to be linked to specific microbes. The dots are yet to be fully joined up, but we do know that maternal diet impacts the microbiome, and that this in turn can lead to poor outcomes, so I don't think it's an unreasonable leap to suggest that eating high amounts of UPF during pre-conception, pregnancy and breastfeeding might be ill-advised. If we're going to cut out swordfish and be wary of herbal teas, we should probably also be thinking twice about industrially made substances, packed with additives, that displace so many nutritious and 'microbiome-feeding' choices from our diet. The impact could be far-reaching, as Toni Harman tried to explain to me: our own maternal microbiome is transmitted to the newborn, and, along with place, mode and timing of birth, type of feeding, environment and geography, affects each baby for a lifetime, during which, if they are female, they will potentially seed the microbes of other future humans... and so on.

Culture vultures

Whilst much remains to be discovered about the human microbiome, and much more still needs to be learnt about the specific and unique female microbiome, there's a good amount of evidence now to support the idea that what we eat impacts our microbiome – and in turn our health – in both positive and negative ways. We've already talked about prebiotics in our discussion of obesity (Chapter 5, page 103) – these are the non-digestible plant cell walls that can help the gut, which in turn can have a positive impact on the health of the rest of our body. If your diet is high in UPF, you won't be eating many prebiotics, for example oats, apples, flaxseeds, leeks, onions, garlic, cashew nuts and almonds. By not eating these sorts of foods, we're not 'feeding' our microbiome anything to ferment to produce those important short chain fatty acids. This can lead to inflammation and, worse still, our hungry microbes may instead use the mucus lining of the gut as a food source instead – *eww!* – eroding it and causing yet more inflammation[25] – which is the driver of so many diseases, from heart disease to arthritis to Parkinson's to depression.[26]

If you've heard about prebiotics, you might also have come across *probiotics*, and the growing trend of eating fermented foods like kombucha, kefir, sauerkraut, kimchi, and even some good old pickles, in order to introduce live bacteria to the gut and improve its microbial variety. In fact, researchers at Stanford University found that eating these foods may have an even more beneficial effect than eating foods high in fibre, increasing diversity and reducing inflammation with dramatic effect in a study they wittily called Fe-Fi-Fo (FErmented & FIbre-rich FOods).[27] There's also been some research into the impact of probiotics on female-specific issues: for example, one study found they improve mood in menopausal women,[28] and another small study scanned the brains of women drinking fermented milk and showed changes in the areas of the brain responsible for processing emotion[29] – clearly much more research is needed. There are many types of fermented food worldwide, as the techniques involved have been used in preserving for centuries. But before we go further, here's a little explainer of some of the most common fermented foods, in case this is not something you've come across. I'm not going to give recipes, as there is a huge wealth of these online, and for many people making these foods at home has become a therapeutic hobby with benefits.

Kombucha: thought to originate in China, kombucha is a slightly fizzy non-alcoholic drink made by fermenting black tea with something called a SCOBY – this stands for Symbiotic Culture of Bacteria and Yeast. The SCOBY is a bit like your sourdough starter, in that you will need to obtain one from a fellow kombucha-maker in order to get going, but once you've got it, your SCOBY will have 'babies' each time you brew.

Sauerkraut: considered a national dish in Germany but perhaps originating from further afield, sauerkraut is made from massaging chopped cabbage with salt, then it's put into a jar where it ferments, releasing its own brine. Said to be a good entry-level project for home fermentation.

Kimchi: originating in Korea and made from Napa cabbage, also known as Chinese cabbage, in a process that to begin with is not a million miles from sauerkraut-making, but which then adds in fiery flavours of ginger, garlic, Korean chilli flakes and fish sauce.

Kefir: fermented milk, for which you'll need 'milk kefir grains'. A bit like your SCOBY, you will have to find a fermenting pal to obtain these from, or purchase online. The grains are sometimes known as the 'seeds of the prophet' and it's said they were a gift to mankind by Muhammed himself – certainly in ancient times their discovery would have brought longevity to milk, a true miracle.

Pickles: if your cucumbers are in vinegar and on a shelf, they're not 'live' or fermented, but if they're in brine – which is just water and salt – they've been through the same process as kimchi and sauerkraut, known as lacto-fermentation. This is when salt wipes out any bad bacteria, allowing the good and friendly lactobacillus to convert any sugars into lactic acid, giving the food that distinctive tang.

These are some of the most common fermented foods that you will hear most about in discussions about eating for health, in particular for the microbiome, but there are others: tempeh, which is a product made from fermented soy beans, apple cider vinegar, sourdough bread, some cheeses (hurrah!) and even Real Ale (double hurrah!). The key feature of all of these foods, and one that distinguishes them hugely from UPF, is that they are essentially everything you want in a lover: fresh, wild, alive and, at times, excitingly unpredictable. In some ways, this is also their downfall: in a world where our palates are used to the bland and unsurprising sugar and salt flavours of UPF, some ferments can seem too challenging, sour and intense. It can take time to adapt to a mindset that says: why go out for McDonald's when you can have kimchi at home?

Something else that's interesting about these fermented foods, when you think about them in the context of UPF, is that they are pretty much impossible to mass produce. You may have had hundreds of UPF-branded biscuits or fast-food burgers over the course of your life, and every single time they are almost exactly the same – in fact, they pride themselves on this global uniformity. Fermented foods cannot be homogenized in this way, they're simply too fresh and feisty. Also, if you buy a product in the shops that claims to be a ferment or tells you it's 'probiotic', proceed with caution. First, if it's kimchi or sauerkraut, for example, and it's not in a fridge, then it's not 'live' – it has been pasteurized and all those microbes are no more. Likewise, if it's a sugary, flavoured ultra-processed yoghurt claiming to be good for your gut, the chances are it's not made in the same way as your homemade kefir – store-bought versions often have the cultures added at the end and are highly regulated for safety reasons, with fermentation having to be halted before bottling to prevent explosions!

Undoubtedly as interest grows in the benefits of these foods there will be more commercially made options on offer, but in this case it does seem like your gut will thank you for making your own or seeking out authenticity. Similarly, you can also consume probiotics by taking supplements – these come in a variety of brands and microbial strains, including some that are specifically marketed at women and claim to support the vaginal microbiome. Some types of probiotic supplements may well have benefits, but trials have shown that they have different effects on different people, sometimes negative.[30] Fermented foods are different from a pill because, as well as probiotics, they also contain prebiotics and 'postbiotics' too, that's the vitamins and nutrients. And, as I've noted as I've researched this book, it's telling that most leading experts on the microbiome seem less interested in supplements than in the big serving of kimchi they're having for lunch.

We need much, much more evidence about the microbiome, and in particular we need to keep reminding researchers to ask, every single time, 'what about the female microbiome?' and 'what about women?', to ensure women's health is not left off the agenda in this momentous and ongoing break-through. In the meantime, there are other ways to improve your microbiome, alongside diet. Having a less clean house and getting a dog are two examples, and as the owner of a small Jack Russell and a rapidly growing and extremely bouncy Labrador puppy, I can confirm that those two are interlinked. In the post-Covid era, we need to stop thinking so 'anti-bacterially' and to question the potential harms of a mindset that says our floors, work surfaces, hands, skin and teeth need to have every micro-organism eradicated. Being in nature is also good but, more importantly, touching it, if you're able, and gardening without gloves, hands in the soil. If you have a garden with enough space, maybe you could even plant a few cabbages for your homemade kimchi? You could become a true fairytale witch, with pots of strange and wonderful plants and cupboards full of bubbling and burping jars. That might be a step too far for some, but it seems like all the evidence shows that wholesome activities that bring us simple pleasure – a walk in the woods, a home-cooked meal, a hug with the dog, planting a few spring bulbs – may all be doing us much more good than we could have ever imagined.

7.

Unlucky women?

Are we too accepting of women's suffering?

Women spend their lives 'under the doctor', as Germaine Greer put it, with so many health issues and corresponding drug treatments associated with being female that you could be forgiven for thinking that being born a woman was 'unlucky' – the biological short straw. Alongside this treatment of the female body as in need of constant medical intervention runs an apparent contradiction: the 'gender knowledge gap'. Essentially, in spite of the fact that there are pills and potions for every single phase of a woman's life, our understanding of women's health is lacking. Women have been, and continue to be left out of research studies, where the male body is treated as the default. Male human subjects, male mice and even male cells tend to be most often used, perhaps due to fears that the cyclical female body will skew results, perhaps due to anxiety over protecting women's fertility, perhaps due to misogyny. Probably, as ever, a mix.

Women grow up with this sense of themselves as outliers, others. We have an inbuilt sense of shame in our bodies, a feeling that they and their functions should be hidden and that, perhaps because of this, we are second best. This does not simply come from the abundance of male mice in research labs, of course, it is ubiquitous in society. We learn it from the most commonly told creation story in the Western world – God is male and Adam was made first and then Eve was made from his rib; we learn it from the dominance of dark suits in group photos of politicians at important summits; we learn it when we are told there are two kinds of football – football, and women's football; we learn it from the power dynamics of our homes, schools and offices. And then we learn it from the cultural messaging around menstruation – the euphemisms, the emphasis on 'hygiene', the tampon wrappers marketed as 'rustle-free'. Whilst this is improving, such subtle cues often still frame periods as a negative and unhygienic experience that we are unfortunately saddled with, rather than as a source of power or pride.

Our experience of female adolescence and of menarche (our first ever period) will together teach us a great deal about what it means to be a woman in our current world. We will then take these lessons forward into matrescence – the phase of life when we transition into mothers (either of children or of ideas and projects, or both), and we meet them again at menopause, sometimes called sagescence, when we change yet again into another version of ourselves, the 'elder' or 'wise woman'.[1] Through all of these life phases Western women are offered the option to be medicalized, and in some cases this is necessary, or even life-saving. But is our perception of the female body as inherently faulty causing us to lean too heavily on this option, and blinding us to the possibility that our health issues may not simply be part of the dreadful package of being female, but exacerbated, or even caused, by other factors that are within our capacity to change? What if we could take back control of our health by changing the way we eat?

I write this chapter in a world in which it's very likely that, if you have one of the health issues mentioned, you have been told by someone – a friend, a relative, or even a health professional – that it's not that serious, or that you are exaggerating, or even that it's probably all in your mind. So I want to be very clear that by making suggestions that diet may be a line of pursuit, I am in no way diminishing or dismissing the very real and serious nature of women's health issues. If you are a woman who has already felt unheard or fobbed off, it could potentially sound glib and insensitive of me to bang on about apples and oily fish. Every woman is different and often it is a combination of standard advice and out-of-the-box thinking that eventually helps. My feeling is that there is very little to lose from giving UPF our focus. But you will know what is best for you. Trust yourself.

First blood

One question I am often asked as the author of a book for pre-teen girls about puberty is, why is the age of first periods younger than it used to be? It's true that this is happening, but 'younger than it used to be' is often doing a lot of heavy lifting in the discussion. The resulting analysis then tends to be oversimplified, based on the current experience of mums in their forties who remember getting their first bra around eleven or twelve and starting their period around thirteen, who now have daughters getting breasts in primary school and starting periods at eleven or twelve. In this sense, yes, the age of menarche is 'younger than it used to be', but the onset of puberty seems to be something quite malleable that has changed quite dramatically in different time periods. In the palaeolithic era, for example, analysis of bone length, which is an indication of oestrogen exposure, has suggested girls started menstruating between the ages of seven and thirteen.[2] But in the mid- to late nineteenth century, periods were starting around age seventeen – and this age has been falling ever since.[3] In fact, since the mid-twentieth century the decline in first period age has slowed down – it's the first signs of puberty, like breasts and pubic hair, that continue to get earlier. So it seems like these changes are complex, and are not just a twenty-first-century phenomenon. Puberty onset and menarche can go up or down, but in response to what?

The answer, as is so often the case with women's health, is 'nobody really knows'. Some suggest connections to the endocrine-disrupting chemicals in our modern world, which are abundant in common items like plastic (in which UPF is often wrapped or contained) and potentially capable of affecting our hormones.[4] Other theories point to the absence of biological fathers or the presence of step-dads and men who are not genetically related in young girls' homes, postulating that this may be causing stress or even some kind of evolutionary imperative to reproduce.[5] But the most widely accepted theories all seem to be focused on one area: rising BMI. With an irony that you couldn't make up, one of the key hormones involved in the onset of puberty, kisspeptin, is named after the ultra-processed chocolate Hershey's Kisses because it was discovered in a lab in Hershey, Pennsylvania. If you have more fat cells, you produce more leptin, and leptin promotes the release of kisspeptin, triggering puberty.

An early start to puberty can not only be distressing, but has also been linked to various health problems, for example mental health issues[6] and a slightly increased risk of breast cancer later in life.[7] While improved nutrition and health probably helped lower the age of puberty in the first half of the twentieth century, it's possible that another nutritional factor is now driving it down further – UPF. We know that UPF is driving obesity and that higher BMI can trigger earlier puberty.[8] However, one study has found that girls who consume lots of drinks with added sugar, like sodas and energy drinks, are likely to start their periods earlier, even when their BMI is lower.[9] A more recent study also found that probiotic yoghurt consumption mitigated the fizzy drink effect on menarche – suggesting the microbiome may be involved.[10] In a 2020 study of over a thousand girls in China, those consuming what researchers call a 'modern dietary pattern' – high in fast foods and low in fibre – were 33 per cent more likely to experience an early menarche than those with the least adherence to this pattern of eating – and, interestingly, this was also independent of their BMI.[11] Another study looked at a Mediterranean diet in nine- and ten-year-olds and found an association with later breast development and menarche, with the authors suggesting more research was needed.[12] We don't have all the evidence yet, but these studies are at least signs that, even in cases of low BMI, what girls are eating has an impact on their age at puberty.

The curse

Once periods have begun, they often bring their own set of problems, the most common being pain. Period pain, or dysmenorrhea as it's officially known, is described as being either 'primary' or 'secondary': in the latter case it's caused by underlying conditions, such as endometriosis or fibroids, but primary dysmenorrhea is simply down to the cramping of the uterus. What the root cause is or why some women have only mild pain whilst others find it debilitating is a question that seems to be mostly surrounded in myth. As a teen, I remember puzzling over it with girlfriends and the only answer we could come up with was 'luck'. During my three pregnancies, I was told several times that because I hadn't had much trouble with painful periods, I would probably find labour contractions easier too. Yet more luck. I do think that, as women, we often accept these vague and unevidenced stories about our bodies unquestioningly, perhaps due to the shocking absence of any real knowledge or information. If we then present to the doctor with our 'unlucky' story of severe period pain, we may find it being dismissed as something women simply have to put up with. Underlying conditions notoriously take a long time to diagnose – 7.5 years in the case of endometriosis – and women often report feeling fobbed off by medical professionals.[13] Another common issue, heavy periods (officially known as menorrhagia), gets similar treatment – they are, according to current NHS advice, 'common and may just be normal for you'.[14] In other words, unlucky.

In fact, both painful and heavy periods do have a cause, even if not related to underlying conditions. Menstrual cramps are caused by prostaglandin, a hormone-like substance that's also responsible for several different functions in the body. But if levels of prostaglandin are too high, this can result in period pain, and can make periods heavier, too. Another factor can be high oestrogen in relation to progesterone, sometimes called 'oestrogen dominance'. The causes for such hormonal imbalances can be complex, and you should always consult your doctor. However, if a medical reason cannot be found, you may find that you are prescribed the contraceptive pill, which, whilst it may be helpful, for example by reducing pain, it does not treat any underlying causes but simply suppresses the menstrual cycle by stopping ovulation. Effectively, any woman taking the pill is masking what the American College of Obstetricians and Gynecologists (ACOG) calls 'the fifth vital sign', meaning it considers menstruation an important indicator of health. Whilst it may not be as important a measure as the other four vital signs – body temperature, pulse, breathing rate and blood pressure – it is certainly worth paying attention to period issues, and perhaps even considering a risk-free potential solution: a change in diet.

Those pain-inducing high prostaglandin levels can be a response to inflammation, which numerous studies have linked to UPF.[15] Some researchers have labelled this inflammation 'fast-food fever', suggesting that the body might not be recognizing UPF as food and mounting an inflammatory response against it.[16] Others suggest the inflammation may be due to additives in UPF that affect the gut microbiome. Still others point to the food that is displaced from our diet when we eat lots of UPF – a Mediterranean diet has been shown to be anti-inflammatory, as has a diet high in omega-3, found in food like oily fish, leafy greens, berries and nuts. Then, of course, there's the impact of diet on the oestrobolome (remember the Sea Witch from our microbiome chapter?! See Chapter 6, page 124). Our gut bacteria may not metabolize oestrogen optimally if we are not eating enough non-digestible plant fibres and a range of other wholefoods. One study of Spanish university students found that those with a low adherence to a Mediterranean diet had longer menstrual cycles, eating less than two pieces of fruit a day made painful periods more likely, and menstrual bleeding was lower in women who consumed olive oil daily.[17] Two separate studies, both conducted before the term UPF was coined or categorized, looked at dietary patterns of women in relation to period pain and found that those eating high levels of 'snacks' and 'junk food' were more likely to have painful periods.[18] All of this points to UPF being something to consider if your periods are painful or heavy, and suggests that far more research needs to be done.

The myth of unluckiness, with its inherent idea that 'you get what you get', may well deter women from seeking solutions, and it may have this same effect on some healthcare professionals too. Two different women got in touch with me during the writing of this book to tell me about how diet affected their experience of pre-menstrual syndrome (PMS) and polycystic ovaries (PCOS). The first, Catherine Oliver, struggled with severe PMS, experiencing 'ten days of exhaustion, severe grumpiness, and sore breasts' each month that made her desperate for her period to start. She didn't consult her doctor because, as she puts it, 'I thought PMT was just a normal, annoying part of being a woman', plus she was keen not to take the contraceptive pill. She then discovered the solution by accident when she stopped eating sugar for Lent, and found her PMS magically evaporated. 'I'm 38 and this means that for nearly half my menstruating life I've felt rubbish the second half of every cycle, which is infuriating,' she told me. 'Although I eat healthily my weakness was sugar, which I now know causes inflammation, meaning my healthy diet wasn't enough to prevent PMT, I needed to cut the sugar out too! I now can't believe how many years I put up with feeling awful and thinking it was just my lot in life.' There is mounting evidence about the role of diet in PMS: one study from 2019 found that diets high in fat, sugar and salt were a risk factor;[19] another from 2020 found that women eating the highest levels of fast food, sodas and processed meats were much more likely to be affected than those eating more traditional diets.[20]

Hannah Wainwright got in touch with me about her experience with PCOS and described how she 'fought for years to be heard by doctors whose only advice was to take the pill, a drug called metformin, or – very unhelpfully in the absence of any specific dietary advice – to simply "lose weight".' Desperate, she sought the help of a nutritionist and changed her diet to wholefoods, largely eliminating UPF. 'This is one of the key things that got me to the point where all my symptoms are either gone or largely under control and my blood tests no longer show any markers for PCOS,' she told me. 'I was privileged to be able to afford to see the nutritionist, but why did the doctor not make dietary suggestions? I was able to regain my health, but this information should be available to every woman at the point of diagnosis.' Research into the relationship between diet and PCOS has begun to focus on UPF – a study in 2022, for example, found that a diet low in UPF 'significantly lowered the odds' of PCOS – but clearly there is much more to learn.[21]

So blessed

Fertility is another female health issue in which luck seems to play an oversized role. The quest to become a mother is one in which some women take on struggles of heroic proportions, ending in the emotional and physical challenge of fertility treatments, whilst others get pregnant simply by hanging their coat up next to their partner's. Some women will then discover an underlying reason why they are struggling to conceive, such as PCOS or endometriosis, whilst others, as many as 30 per cent, will be told their issues are 'unexplained'. Of course, it takes two to tango, and in up to half of cases the cause may be the male partner's sperm. There are already some studies into the impact of UPF on semen: research in 2024 found that replacing 10 per cent of energy from UPF with 10 per cent of energy from unprocessed or minimally processed food was associated with a higher total sperm count, improved sperm motility (that's the ability to travel) and normal sperm forms;[22] another study in 2022 also found that high UPF consumption negatively affected motility even when adjusting for other factors like age, BMI and lifestyle.[23]

Other studies prior to the categorization of UPF are also interesting: two separate pieces of research found that a high consumption of processed red meats (defined as items like hot dogs, burgers, bacon and salami) was associated with low sperm quality and less successful IVF treatment, whereas eating chicken or fish improved fertility;[24] another in 2008 found a relationship between 'soy foods' and semen quality – and on the list of 'soy foods' are plenty of meat and dairy substitutes, ready meals and energy bars, in other words, UPF.[25] Globally, it's thought that sperm count has been declining since the mid-twentieth century, and some experts see a direct relationship between this timing and the advent of a modern processed diet.[26] Other key factors getting the blame are obesity,[27] along with the chemicals found in plastics,[28] and the microplastics that are now everywhere in our world.[29] When researching this, I couldn't help thinking about those supermarket 'Valentine's Day Meal Deals' and how, wrapped in plastic and stuffed with soy, sugar and fat, they might have some hidden contraceptive value (whether we like it or not).

In the female body, the effects of diet on fertility seem clear, and yet women report that this is often not mentioned to them when they seek help. 'I was only told to cut out coffee,' one woman told me. 'They told me to keep stress low and take Vitamin D and folic acid,' said another. 'I changed my diet, but only because I did my own research,' reported one woman who went on to conceive at forty years of age. An experienced former NHS fertility nurse I spoke to, Erica Spooner, admitted, 'Not enough time is spent talking about diet. Women are often simply told to "lose weight" which can be extremely difficult if you have PCOS or are miserable due to your struggle to conceive.' Even before the discussion began about UPF, there was plenty of evidence that a diet high in trans fats,[30] sugar and refined carbohydrates (all typical of UPF) can negatively affect female fertility, and that eating a more 'Mediterranean' diet, high in plant fibre and protein, omega-3 fatty acids, etc., could have a positive impact.[31]

As we saw in Chapter 6, there is also growing evidence that diet impacts the gut and vaginal microbiomes and that this in turn may impact our ability to conceive or our chance of miscarriage, as well as playing a role in conditions such as endometriosis and PCOS that can also make getting pregnant more difficult. Obesity, too, which we know is directly related to UPF consumption, can also cause menstrual issues, reduced ovulation and infertility.[32] And one 2018 study found that women eating less fruit and more 'fast food' whilst trying to conceive was associated with taking a longer time to get pregnant.[33] It seems surprising, then, that women report that diet is not given more focus in their appointments about fertility issues. One wonders cynically whether this could be simply because, whilst the global fertility industry is worth millions of dollars, there is not a great deal of profit to be made out of suggesting people ditch the Valentine's meal deals and try a homemade chicken supreme instead. And whilst there aren't any studies as yet into the specific effect of UPF on libido, there are plenty that look at the positive impact of healthy eating on everything from mood, which can affect libido,[34] to the blood flow to our genitals, increasing female arousal.[35] One, albeit slightly tenuous, study even found that an apple a day improved women's sex lives, perhaps due to the polyphenols and antioxidants – maybe Eve was on to something.[36]

Respect to the X

It's thought that one in ten people globally are now affected by an autoimmune disorder – in which the immune system wrongly attacks healthy parts of the body as if they were foreign or harmful.[37] Of those affected by autoimmune disorders, the majority – around 80 per cent – are women. Every single autoimmune condition is more prevalent in females, and in some, extremely so. Lupus, for example, which causes extreme tiredness, joint pain and a rash on the face, is around nine times more prevalent in women than men. Sjogren's syndrome, which affects parts of the body that produce fluids causing dryness, has a female to male ratio of 19:1. Scientists are still trying to understand these disorders, the numbers of which began rising globally around four decades ago, but it's currently thought that the reason they attack women in far higher numbers is down to the fact that while men have one X and one Y chromosome, women have a double helping of X.

The story of chromosomes and how they are perceived is shot through with the sexism that has forever been endemic in science. For starters, the woman who first observed chromosomes, Nettie Stevens, was sidelined by male colleagues who took most of the credit for her work. Then, the idea that women had XX whereas men had XY was somehow spun as a negative for women, with the idea being widely held that the second X was surplus to requirements and therefore 'switched off'. Tales were then told about the great advantage of the Y, that magical extra that we unlucky women lacked: 'There was always an incessant buzz about the Y chromosome because most of the people speaking breathlessly about it had one as well,' as Sharon Moalem puts it in his book, *The Better Half: On the Genetic Superiority of Women*. In fact, the 'extra' X is not 'switched off', and not all genes in it are inactivated. Rather, it provides women with an advantage, backing up our immune system and explaining why we are tougher than men from cradle to grave, being more likely to survive premature birth, disease, traumatic injury, adversity and famine, across the board.

This is thought by some to be an evolutionary feature, ensuring women's survival during their childbearing years and enabling them to live to protect their young and therefore the species.[38] But this immune advantage is a double-edged sword because these immune cells, which use genes to recognize and attack viruses, have effectively twice the chance of misfiring an attack on the wrong target, making females so much more susceptible to autoimmune disease.[39] Some of the slowness of discovery on this science is also part of the sexism story: using only male mice and male cell lines, for example, has meant that researchers have missed the unique genetic complexities of the female immune response.[40]

Autoimmune conditions are triggered by an interplay between genes and environment – you may be more genetically susceptible, but your lifestyle also plays a part, explaining why, in some cases, one identical twin but not the other will develop an autoimmune disorder. But since human genetic make-up hasn't changed in the past few decades, something else must have changed.[41] James Lee, a world expert in autoimmune disorders based at the Francis Crick Institute in London, told me: 'We don't know specifically what's changed in the last forty years that has caused a rise in autoimmune diseases, and it's likely a combination of factors – pollution, obesity, stress, early-life antibiotics, infections – but our Western diet is likely a contributing factor, for example emulsifiers in our food could thin the protective mucus in our guts and bring our microbiomes into direct contact with our immune systems.'

A 2024 study by researchers at Harvard University looked at the diets of over 200,000 women, with more than twenty years of follow-up, and found that those consuming the highest amount of UPF were over 50 per cent more likely to develop lupus than those in the group consuming the least amount of UPF.[42] Several studies have shown a link between high consumption of UPF and Inflammatory Bowel Disease (IBD), with particularly strong findings for Crohn's disease, the type of IBD that women are most likely to have.[43]

One study found that women with fibromyalgia, an autoimmune disorder that causes pain and tenderness all over the body, as well as fatigue and insomnia, reported an improvement in symptoms, including less pain and better sleep, after following a three-month anti-inflammatory diet that included cutting out UPF.[44] Another smaller study found that women who cut out monosodium glutamate (MSG) and aspartame had 'complete, or almost complete resolution' of their fibromyalgia symptoms.[45] If you're female, you're three times more likely than a man to suffer from rheumatoid arthritis (RA), where the immune system wrongly attacks the cells that line your joints, and research has found that a Western diet may increase your risk of RA by boosting inflammation or by increasing insulin resistance and obesity.[46] If you have RA, you're also at as much as a 70 per cent increased risk of cardiovascular disease, and here again research has found that a diet low in UPF can reduce this specific risk in RA sufferers.[47] And an Italian study in 2023 found that high consumption of UPF worsened the severity of symptoms in multiple sclerosis (MS) sufferers.[48]

All of these autoimmune diseases have also been linked to gut dysbiosis, when the species of bacteria in our microbiomes are out of balance or less diverse than they should be.[49] How our colonies of microbes are potentially being changed by UPF or specific food additives is still unravelling. A series of research by Aaron Lerner, a professor at Tel Aviv University, and German researcher Torsten Matthias has looked at the impact of an additive called transglutaminase on coeliac disease, an autoimmune disorder in which the immune system attacks your tissues when you eat gluten, and which affects two to three times more women than men. Researching this, I made some discoveries that shocked me. Transglutaminase is also known as 'meat glue', and it's used to make those 'reformed' types of meat you are probably familiar with. They're sometimes jokingly called 'Frankenmeats' because they are basically lots of scraps of meat, sometimes mechanically reclaimed, stuck together with meat glue and then wrapped in plastic and shaped into what look like cuts of meat, but actually aren't. I guess that although I tried not to think about this, I did know it happened, but what I didn't know was that transglutaminase or meat glue is an ingredient that is considered a 'processing aid' and therefore doesn't have to appear on the list of food ingredients, even in the UK. Lerner and Matthias's research looked at meat glue and found it a 'likely culprit' in the development of coeliac disease and a 'potential public health concern'. They found that meat glue – used in a variety of foods, including chicken nuggets, yoghurt, meatballs, hot dogs, tofu and sushi – along with six other food additives, weakened the 'tight junctions' in the gut, causing bacteria and toxins to leak into the system and the body to mount an immune response. Based on their findings, they suggested that anyone with a family history of autoimmune conditions avoid UPF.[50]

Does my vagina look big in this?

Nowhere in the female lifespan does the idea that being a woman is a terrible bit of bad luck become more vivid than during pregnancy and childbirth. I've written extensively about this life experience, trying to reframe it and encourage people to talk and think about it more positively, but it has been an uphill struggle. It's so engrained in all of us, from film and TV and the horror stories we hear, to fear childbirth and to see it as a sort of disaster from which we need to be rescued. It's very common for women themselves to expect their bodies to be incapable of birthing or to blame their bodies when their births don't go according to plan. It's rare for it to be acknowledged that the system in which women have their babies is not serving women well, and that their birth stories could be less traumatic and more positive if simple things were implemented, like continuity of care (that's every woman having the chance to build a relationship with her midwife and know and trust the person who is by her side in labour). It was this 'fix the system, not the women' argument that I was trying to make in a discussion about rising caesarean rates on BBC Radio Scotland back in 2019, with a doctor who was on to make the opposing argument (presumably, 'fix the women, not the system', a line it always baffles me that people are willing to take). And just as our on-air discussion was drawing to a close, he made an extraordinary claim – he stated that obesity was causing women to have a build-up of fat tissue in their birth canal, making it narrower and more difficult for the baby to get out. In other words, the blame for increasingly medicalized births lay with women, and their fat vaginas.

This is categorically untrue, but it does work well in our woman-blaming culture: rather than doing anything to change or improve childbirth, it's much easier to just say that it's women's fault for having babies when they're old and fat (rather than slim and tied to the kitchen sink straight out of college, just like in the good old days!). However, while it's false to say that women are to blame for all the current difficult and traumatic births, and it's *definitely* false to say that babies are struggling to get out of fat vaginas (the vagina is an internal muscle and will be pretty much the same whatever your weight), there *are* increased health risks to women with obesity in pregnancy, for example gestational diabetes, miscarriage, high blood pressure and pre-eclampsia.[51] You may also have a more difficult birth, perhaps because you are less mobile, or perhaps because other health issues will mean a more medicalized experience in which your choices are restricted, for example you might find you are told you are 'not allowed' to give birth in the midwife-led birth centre or have a water birth. So whilst it's important to acknowledge that being overweight or obese in pregnancy (which can be related to a diet higher in UPF) is probably not serving women well, it's important that we don't use women's body size as a scapegoat for everything that's wrong with the current maternity system. Dr Alice Keely is 'The Heavyweight Midwife' and specializes in positive birth experiences for plus-size women. She told me:

> 'The risks of being overweight in pregnancy are complex and are often over-simplified by health professionals. They tend to distil complexity down to the catch-all 'high risk', which suggests that weight-associated pregnancy complications are 'likely', when they absolutely are not. Many pregnant women are referred for unwanted dietary advice, which stigmatizes and patronizes them. Many women also struggle with weight gain and retention throughout their lives, and the reasons are known to be psychologically complex. Plus-size pregnant women should be cared for with respect and dignity and offered full support for their birth choices, and also reassured that any increased risks due to their weight are very small.

The key for all women is to be listened to and get really good-quality personalized care.'

Just as some people (and I was one of them) use pregnancy as the motivation they need to quit smoking, the time when you are thinking about starting a family is probably a good moment to cut down or cut out UPF, regardless of your weight, and there's mounting evidence to support you in that decision. A huge meta-analysis of all the data on a diet high in UPF in pregnancy found an increased risk of gestational diabetes and pre-eclampsia in all women who ate this way, not just those living with overweight or obesity.[52] Both of these conditions will mean women being given the label of 'high risk' and therefore being more likely to have a more medicalized birth, which can be less satisfying and potentially more traumatic. Another large-scale research analysis, a collaboration between Tommy's National Centre for Miscarriage Research and the University of Birmingham in 2023, looked at the data from over 63,000 women and found that a diet high in UPF was associated with double the risk of miscarriage – but that a high intake of fruit and vegetables saw a similar risk reduction.[53] Two separate studies have found that eating high levels of UPF in what they call the 'periconceptional period' – that's the time from shortly before you get pregnant and into the pregnancy itself – is associated with smaller embryonic growth,[54] with the second study worryingly finding an association with impaired head circumference.[55]

Some studies seem to show that it's the increased exposure to phthalates (pronounced THA-lates) in the plastic that wraps so much UPF that is at least part of the problem – these chemical compounds are thought to disrupt the endocrine system and possibly increase the risk of low birth weight and pre-term birth. Several animal studies have shown that exposure to phthalates in the first trimester is associated with shorter anogenital distance (AGD) in males (the distance between the anus and base of the penis) and one study in humans has had similar findings, although more research is needed.[56] This reduced AGD has implications for future fertility. A 2022 study found an association between higher maternal consumption of UPF and shorter AGD, postulating that this could be due to the lower intake of key nutrients, but also suggesting a possible link with UPF and phthalates exposure.[57] And a study published in February 2024 found higher levels of phthalates in the urine of pregnant women whose diets were high in UPF.[58]

There are a raft of 'soda studies' into soft drink consumption in pregnancy. Before we go any further into them, it's worth remembering that, generally, in terms of diet, pregnant women are not advised to take even the most miniscule of risks. For example, the chance of getting listeria from eating unpasteurized blue cheese is thought to be around 1 in 8,000, and even if you are in that unlucky 0.01 per cent, the chance that your baby will suffer harm is even smaller again. Nevertheless, we all lay off the Roquefort in pregnancy, along with a long list of other food and drink items in a general spirit of 'better safe than sorry'. With sodas, however, there are no official warnings, which is surprising given that they are absolutely surplus to requirements in our diet and numerous studies have highlighted risks. A large study in

2010 of nearly 60,000 Danish women found an association between artificially sweetened sodas and pre-term birth,[59] and a further large study in 2012 found this risk association extended to fizzy drinks that are sweetened with sugar, too.[60] Another study found an association between caffeinated soft drinks in pregnancy and cerebral palsy risk.[61] Another two suggest a link between maternal soda consumption and the development of asthma;[62] another between sugar-sweetened soft drinks and the risk of congenital heart defects in the baby.[63] None of these findings is definitive and more research is needed. It's almost certainly true that the odd fizzy drink in pregnancy is unlikely to cause harm, but then, neither is the odd helping of pâté or glass of wine, and most women fastidiously avoid them.

There are other studies that focus on UPF more generally in pregnancy. One looking at pregnant women in Brazil found that high UPF consumption itself led to oxidative stress,[64] associated not just with autism but with several other adverse outcomes, including miscarriage, pre-eclampsia, fetal growth restriction and pre-term labour.[65] Other studies suggest a longer-term impact on the baby, for example one found an association between a maternal diet high in UPF and verbal functioning in childhood, which is an important measure of neurodevelopment,[66] and another found that the child of a mother with a high UPF diet had an increased risk of being overweight or obese, and this was independent of any lifestyle risk factors.[67] Whilst pregnant women don't need more stuff to feel anxious or guilty about, they do need clear information and evidence, and it would seem that the reduction of UPF during pregnancy is something that we should be giving more focus.

From cradle to grave we women are taught to believe that to be female is to suffer; from the pain and inconvenience of periods, to the burden of pregnancy, to the horrors of menopause, our bodies are blamed for everything. Part of the solution to this lies in calling out a medical system that simultaneously pathologizes the female body and fails to properly understand it. When I spoke to Ina Schuppe Koistinen, Associate Professor at the Karolinska Institutet in Sweden, about the vaginal microbiome, she put it to me quite succinctly: 'The stark contrast between the millions spent on researching erectile dysfunction and the chronic underfunding of women's health is staggering. It's a clear reflection of societal priorities – while billions have been invested in solving one very specific issue, conditions like endometriosis, PCOS and the vaginal microbiome, affecting millions of women, remain critically under-researched. It's time we recognized that women's health deserves at least the same level of attention and funding.' We need to keep calling for this to happen, but while we wait for systemic change, it seems we could potentially make a big, positive impact on many of the conditions we accept as just part of the raw deal of being female, simply by turning our back on UPF.

8.

I'll have the blues

Depression on the menu

As a writer, I have to remind myself constantly about the relationship between my gut and my brain. Bringing a book to life on the page takes a certain amount of tenacity; you need the ability to sit there when the word count is 273 and keep going, knowing you've got another 4,727 to go until you've even come close to something worthy of being called a 'chapter'. And that you've then got to repeat that until you've got twelve chapters. During this process, there are many highs and lows, probably more lows than highs if I'm truly honest. There's plenty of self-doubt, imposter syndrome and wishing you'd been better at maths and embarked on a lucrative career in accounting. But sometimes this really comes to a head and you find yourself thinking, 'I'm useless, nobody is ever going to read this, it's all a big pile of crap, I can't do it, I'm stupid, I give up.' Over the years, though, I've discovered a pattern to this existential crisis – it happens daily, at around 11.42 a.m. And it has a simple solution: lunch.

Although I know this scenario well, I do still have to 'mother' myself at these times and almost frog-march myself unwillingly to the fridge to fix up a sandwich. Because even though it happens often and three bites into my cheese and crackers I'm already feeling completely different, when I'm fully in the throes of the 'why-did-you-ever-think-you-could-write-a-book?' negative spiral, it does actually seem completely real to me and not related to food in the slightest. In fact, it took me until I was in my late thirties to even start to be able to acknowledge the relationship between hunger and my emotional state. Before that, I just flailed around, wondering why all my life problems seemed to mysteriously come to a head at noon. One thing that helped me to make the link was the sudden widespread use of the word 'hangry', used to describe that mix of hunger and anger that, when you're in the midst of it, definitely feels like it's 100 per cent down to the fact that you're surrounded by idiots and absolutely zero to do with food. The following social media meme also woke me up to the idea that, although it's important to take our feelings seriously, it's always worth taking a moment to consider whether they are simply manifestations of basic needs not being met.

If you feel like you hate everyone: eat.
If you feel like everyone hates you: sleep.
If you feel like you hate yourself: shower.
If you feel like everyone hates everyone: go outside.

Simple – but it should probably be taught in schools. The fact is we're just not very good at making the connection between our body and our mind, so accustomed are we to thinking of them as two separate entities. This is probably not our fault – a few centuries of mind-body dualism have ensured that most of us think of our thoughts and emotions as a sort of floaty entity carried about by our more earthy and practical bodies. Even if we acknowledge that we do sometimes get a bit tetchy or overwhelmed when we need a snack, it's second nature for most of us to assume that what we eat really only has an impact on our physical health. Mental health is something different – definitely not affected by diet, right? When you think about it, it's odd that we think this. Most of us will readily swallow an antidepressant tablet and confidently expect it to have an impact on how we feel, and yet it doesn't occur to us that something else that we swallow – food – might have similar powers. An emerging field of science has begun to explore this impact: nutritional psychology. Cutting-edge research over the past decade has demonstrated that what we eat can play a powerful role in our mental health.[1] It would be great if the current medical model would begin to consider the role of diet a little more – we are still in a place where a visit to the doctor with depression is unlikely to involve many questions about what you are eating. And if you're a woman, it's also possible that your difficulties will be further compounded by the engrained cultural assumption that the real problem is something rather fundamental that can't be treated, not even by food: your femaleness.

All in her head

The history of women's mental health has been shot through with appalling misogyny since the dawn of time. Or at least since a flipping long time ago – we don't have a record of what Early Man decided was amiss with Early Woman, of course, but we do know that as long ago as 1900 BC the Ancient Egyptians were already putting women's distress down to the uterus moving around within the body. The Greeks took a similar line, coming up with theories about curative sex that still echo today, along the lines of, 'what she needs is a good seeing to'.

Hippocrates first came up with the term 'hysteria' in the fifth century BC, suggesting, like the Egyptians, that any woman with any kind of unexplained complaint must have a 'wandering womb', the cure for which was inhalation of aromatic herbs and fumigation of the genitals and – you've guessed it – marriage and sex. These ideas were continued by the Romans, who only disagreed on whether the better cure was lots of sex or no sex at all. In the Middle Ages, the idea that women were somehow 'defective', begun by Ancients like Aristotle, who saw women as 'deformed males', began to take an even stronger hold, helped by thinkers such as Thomas Aquinas who helpfully proposed that 'the woman is a failed man'. As Christianity became increasingly powerful, this female 'defectiveness' evolved into something more sinister – the idea of woman as 'witch', possessed by the Devil, and her mental illness or 'hysteria' seen as evidence of her sin and sorcery. Women, responsible for the Fall itself, were less Godly than men and treated with great suspicion, in particular if they were old, opinionated, unhappy or unwell with an illness that could not be explained. Such women were surely possessed, and were burned at the stake in their thousands.

The witch hunts eventually stopped, but the idea of hysteria and female defectiveness pervaded, all the way through to the Victorians – whose smelling salts were a nod to Hippocrates' ideas of pungent odours returning the womb to its place – and then on to Freud – whose ideas still contained remnants of sex (with a man, of course!) as a treatment for mental ill health, and positioned females as the lesser and yet more manipulative and deceitful sex. In the twentieth century, women were imprisoned in mental hospitals for their challenges to patriarchy in the form of sex outside of marriage or lack of compliance, in the same way they were once burned for similar reasons. Hysteria was not removed from the *Diagnostic Statistical Manual* (DSM, used by mental health professionals) until 1980.[2] And even today, women report their mental ill health being dismissed as a manifestation of their female weakness: a 2023 survey from the charity Campaign against Living Miserably (CALM) found that one in five women who sought help for their mental health were told they were being 'dramatic'; a third were asked if they were 'overthinking things'; 20 per cent were asked if they were on their period; and 27 per cent were told their issues could be hormonal.[3] These systemic attitudes prevent women from seeking help for mental health issues, say CALM, with over a quarter of the women surveyed saying they fear they won't be taken seriously, or will be labelled 'attention-seeking' or 'over-emotional'.[4]

In the context of this history, discussing the possible impact of diet on women's mental health could be seen as insensitive – simply replacing, 'what you need is more sex', with, 'what you need is more broccoli, luv'. So it's important to be clear – mental health issues like depression are very real and they are multi-factorial. Adverse childhood experiences (ACEs), for example, are known to increase the likelihood of depression, as do other factors such as difficult life circumstances, or a family history of depressive illness. Anyone struggling with mental ill health needs holistic support, but when you look at the evidence, as we will do in this chapter, it seems like information about the possible impact of diet should be a much bigger consideration than it is currently. And women need this information more than anyone because one of the biggest risk factors for depression is your sex – if you're female, you are twice as likely to suffer it.

We don't yet have an explanation for why this is. It has been suggested that it could be due to our hormonal cycles or that there could be a social element, since women are more likely to experience abuse or violence, to live in poverty, or to be carers. Scientists have historically avoided studying depression in females due to the potential unpredictability introduced by the effects of the menstrual cycle.[5] But while restricting studies to males may have made their research easier to conduct, it has almost certainly made women's lives more difficult. Depression in women, still so poorly understood, is now the leading cause of disease burden in women worldwide,[6] and rates are rising: over one-third of women in the USA now report having been diagnosed with it at least once in their lifetime, and the rate for women has been rising at nearly twice the rate for men since 2017.[7]

Whilst more men than women die by suicide, around twice as many women attempt it. The numbers are shocking – in the USA the suicide rate among women is described as 'soaring', with, for example, increases of 80–90 per cent in young and middle-aged women between 1999 and 2017.[8] In the UK in 2021, nearly four women a day took their own lives;[9] every two days, one of those women was under 25.[10]

The reasons for these terrible figures are complex and, as we shall see in this chapter, poor mental health is often part of a variety of vicious cycles that overlap, grow and spiral in ways that can seem overwhelmingly hard to address. But whether we want to make changes at a social and political level, or in our own lives, the growing evidence on UPF offers a clear opportunity for breakthrough: start with the food on your plate.

Standard American Diet = SAD

The next time you tuck into a UPF feast of burgers, fries, and Coke with a factory-made cake for dessert, otherwise known as the Standard American Diet, remember what it stands for: SAD. For some time now, researchers have been finding stronger and stronger evidence that this way of eating has an impact on our emotional health as well as our physical bodies. A study published in September 2023 looked at the diets and mental health of over 31,000 women between the ages of 42 and 62, and found that women who ate the most UPF – nine servings per day – were 50 per cent more likely to develop depression than those who ate the least, i.e. no more than four servings a day.[11] This study was important because not only did they adjust the data for other risk factors of depression, such as age, BMI and socio-economic status, they also assessed the women's diets years before the onset of depression, thus ruling out the possibility that the study subjects were eating UPF because they were depressed, rather than vice versa. When the researchers drilled into the data, they also found a really strong association between one particular UPF ingredient and depression onset – artificial sweeteners. The reason for this link is not yet fully understood, but Dr Andrew Chan, one of the study's co-authors, has suggested that chronic inflammation, and also the role of the gut microbes, both require further consideration.[12]

An umbrella review in 2024 – when researchers look at the commonalities in the findings of lots of studies – also found a link to the artificial sweetener aspartame, and concluded there was a significant association between overall UPF consumption and depression.[13] They suggested that this may be because of the nutritional quality of UPF – high in fat, salt and sugar, and low in fibre, micronutrients and phytochemicals such as polyphenols (healthy compounds found in plants) – causing inflammation or oxidative stress. Chemicals like aspartame in UPF may be adding to the problem by inhibiting the release of neurotransmitters like dopamine and serotonin, both of which play roles in feelings of pleasure and happiness. One 2022 study of mice found that aspartame produced anxiety-like behaviour, and that this anxiety then appeared in the mice's descendants.[14] This study was conducted on male mice, and mice, of course, are not humans. But given that the WHO has raised concerns that aspartame, albeit in high quantities, may be 'possibly carcinogenic to humans', it would seem like assuming the worst about this ingredient is the best approach.

Other research has looked at the impact of diet on the mental health of both pregnant women and their offspring. A 2024 study into pregnant women in Brazil found that those with a high consumption of UPF had higher levels of anxiety, stress, depressive symptoms and feelings of sadness.[15] A different study, the NUTRIMUM trial in New Zealand, found that giving pregnant women micronutrient tablets – broad spectrum vitamins and minerals – during pregnancy greatly improved symptoms of antenatal depression and also had a positive impact on their babies, who in follow-up studies displayed better emotional regulation and fewer signs of stress.[16] And another study, this time in France in 2021, found that adherence to a healthy diet in pregnancy reduced the likelihood of depression and anxiety in children.[17] To date, there have been no studies specifically on UPF and post-natal depression (PND), although there have been several showing that a Mediterranean diet[18] or 'health-conscious diet'[19] reduces the risk of suffering PND, and that a Western diet, high in processed meat, makes it more likely.[20]

Given the prevalence of mental ill health in women, all research into UPF and depression is highly relevant to us. The analysis published in the *British Medical Journal* in February 2024 into the impact of UPF on all areas of health found that a diet high in UPF was associated with a 22 per cent increased risk of depression, particularly in those whose diet comprises at least 30 per cent UPF.[21] Several other studies have reported similar findings,[22] with one concluding that those consuming UPF several times a day are three times more likely to have serious mental health struggles.[23] Another, from a team of Brazilian researchers that included Carlos Monteiro, who developed the Nova scale, found that every 10 per cent increase in the proportion of UPF in the diet was associated with a 10 per cent greater chance of depressive symptoms.[24] Another huge study of over 20,000 people in France, known as NutriNet-Santé, looked almost exclusively at women and again found that, even when removing confounding factors, the more UPF in the diet, the higher the depression risk.[25]

Often such studies are what is known as 'prospective' – this means they look at how UPF in the diet may lead to depression over time. But another important study, known as the SMILEs trial (Supporting the Modification of lifestyle in Lowered Emotional States), did something different.[26] It took people who already had depression and explored whether changing their diet would alleviate their symptoms. Participants, over 70 per cent of whom were women, all had major depression and all were eating a poor-quality diet, high in UPF. They were split into two groups. Both groups were offered something called 'befriending', where they met with a researcher for regular social support. But only one group received a dietary intervention, receiving help and information to follow a largely Mediterranean diet. By the end of the study, the results were hugely impactful: a third of those in the dietary support group met criteria for remission of major depression, compared to

8 per cent of those in the social support group. The more participants adhered to the diet, the greater the improvements they experienced. As an interesting aside, researchers found the high UPF diet to be the more expensive of the two.

Gut feelings

The question of why the amount of UPF in our diet has this powerful impact on our mental health, in particular on symptoms of depression, is not yet fully answered. As always with UPF, the question remains: is it about the unhealthy food we *are* eating, or the healthy food we are *not* eating, or a combination of both? There is plenty of good evidence that a healthy diet can improve our mental health, and even studies that suggest it could reduce our risk of self-harm and suicide,[27] and we also know that if we're eating a lot of UPF, this probably means that many of the foods with their polyphenols and micronutrients and fibres beneficial for our health are *not* being eaten. And it's not just us who are missing out – there's a whole colony of disappointed microbes in our guts that are not getting the foods they need and crave, which means, in turn, that we are also depriving our brains. What we eat is part of our fundamental two-way relationship with our gut microbiome; as we feed them, they produce compounds, many of which are building-blocks for some of the most important brain-signalling molecules, such as dopamine and serotonin. Added to this, our gut microbes play a role in manufacturing short chain fatty acids via their metabolic activity, and these are thought to play a key part in the signals between our gut and brain.[28] The very structure and function of our brains, and thus our mental and emotional states and our outward behaviour, are all influenced by the food we send down for our resident microbes to chew on. Not enough fibre or micronutrients from plants and legumes and your gut microbes will definitely be underperforming; too many UPF additives like emulsifiers, colours and sweeteners may also have a negative impact, disrupting signals between gut and brain.

Interestingly, people who have poor dental health are more likely to have depression[29] and the oral microbiome – which is, of course, also a part of our digestive system – is thought to have a role, which is still being explored.[30] One theory is that it's the hormone cortisol, present in elevated levels in saliva when we are stressed or anxious, that is causing damage both to our teeth and to our gut microbes. Another suggestion is that bacteria from the mouth could be crossing the 'blood-brain barrier' (BBB), triggering an immune response and the neuroinflammation that is associated with mental ill health. Researchers are also beginning to map the differing microbes in the guts of people with a variety of mental health issues, and finding that each disorder has its own specific colony, with some, like schizophrenia and bipolar disorder, seeming to have species that are unique to people with these diagnoses.[31] It seems extraordinary to think that you could tell a person's mental health diagnosis by looking at their microbes, but whether these changes are due to diet, medication, or the disease itself is not yet known. And, in the case of depression, researchers have even found that there are differences in the microbiomes of people according to their sex, with the species of gut microbes in women with major depression differing not just from other people without depression, but from the gut microbes of depressed men.[32] A study conducted in Spain in 2021 looked at the diversity and composition of the microbiome in people consuming five or more servings of UPF a day and found that, even when consuming the same quantity and type of UPF, the microbiota in women was different from that in men.[33] They also found that the incidence of depression and anxiety was higher in people consuming such amounts, particularly female participants.

Psychobiotics

The idea that bacteria can be used therapeutically, a field known as psychobiotics, is also gaining an evidence base.[34] Psychobiotics began with the observation that people who lived in communities that ate high levels of fermented foods tended to live longer. Now researchers are exploring the idea of giving people particular strains of bacteria, or cocktails of different strains, and assessing changes in their mental health. In a study on post-natal depression, for example, over 200 women were randomly assigned either a strain of bacteria called *Lactobacillus rhamnosus* HN001 or a placebo, during their pregnancy and for six months following the birth. The women receiving HN001 reported significantly less depression and anxiety than those in the placebo group.[35] In other studies, menopausal women with symptoms like depression and mood swings have been helped by psychobiotics, although more research is needed.[36]

Perhaps our rapidly developing knowledge of the microbiome will eventually hold the key to the much higher rates of particular types of mental ill health in women – for now, we can only say that it's a priority for women to think about ways to be attentive to their gut, and diet is a key way to do this. Experts agree: Ted Dinan, Professor of Psychiatry at University College Cork and a leading expert on the gut-brain axis, told me: 'In the future, we will definitely see psychobiotics being used to treat milder forms of depression and anxiety. In the meantime, our modern diet is almost certainly contributing to our 'missing microbes', which could mean we're dealing with stress less effectively. There's a simple solution: eat more plants.'

Something fishy

Another important factor in depression is inflammation, which is something that is meant to happen in our bodies as a response to infection, injury or illness.[37] You will see inflammation in action if you cut yourself, for example, as redness, heat and swelling arrive at the area in need of healing. But part of this essential action is that, once the problem is fixed, the inflammation 'switches off'. To do this, the body needs, in particular, an omega-3 fatty acid known as DHA, found in fish and seafood. A diet high in UPF could be described as an 'inflammatory' diet, perhaps because our bodies treat some elements of UPF not as food but as foreign bodies, mounting an immune response to their presence, or perhaps because of the anti-inflammatory foods that we miss out on when we eat UPF, in particular the omega-3 fatty acids we gain from oily fish.[38] And the chronic inflammation this diet may cause is thought to play a substantial role in depression, by disrupting neurotransmitters, reducing brain neuroplasticity that enables us to adapt, and even by inflaming the brain itself. A 2023 study, in which 70 per cent of participants were female, found that taking an omega-3 supplement alongside standard anti-depressant medication significantly reduced the severity of the depression;[39] other studies have recommended omega-3 supplements in the treatment and prevention of postnatal depression.[40] A large study in France in 2019 found that a pro-inflammatory diet – of high sugar and fat, refined grains and processed meats – increased the likelihood of depression in women specifically.[41] Several other studies have had similar findings: the Standard American Diet seems to be making women sad, more than it is men.[42] Why?

Could the answer lie with inflammation? The female body is more prone to inflammation because of our second X chromosome (this is also why we are much more likely to suffer from autoimmune conditions,[43] see page 152). Are our bodies mounting an immune response to something in UPF? People who have had adverse childhood experiences (ACEs), such as abuse, are also more disposed towards chronic inflammation,[44] and women report more ACEs than men and are far more likely to be sexually abused. We are told that women then tend to 'turn inwards' with their feelings, becoming depressed, whereas their male counterparts 'turn outwards' with behaviours like drug-taking or aggression. But could it be that the reasons lie in physical differences rather than emotional ones – something in our genes, or our microbiome? At the moment, we just don't know.

One thing is clear: anti-inflammatory foods, which you are unlikely to be eating much of in a high UPF diet, seem key in reducing depression risk. These foods include fibre direct from unprocessed plants (with their intact 'matrix'), garlic, ginger and turmeric, and – again, really important this one – oily fish and seafood. One academic, Professor Michael Crawford at Imperial College London, has spent the last five decades warning people of the impact of a lack of fish in the diet on the brain, particularly in the maternal diet,[45] and believes that not just our mental health but even our IQ is declining as a result.[46] He suggests that human beings only evolved to be of such high intelligence – in comparison to other mammals – because of their consumption of fish, the richest source of DHA.[47] Much simpler to catch than a meaty land mammal, our ancestors would have delighted in the fruits of rivers, lakes and the sea, scooping out shellfish and netting fish with relative ease. His words to me were stark: 'The decline in mental health and IQ can only be reversed by attention to maternal nutrition before and during pregnancy with the provision of proper foods that support brain health. The continued decline can only end in extinction.' Women need to start putting mackerel, shellfish and, if the budget will stretch, salmon back onto their plates, or start taking a supplement – for their own mental health, that of their possible offspring and, if Professor Crawford is right, the future of the human race.

Vicious cycles

So, what we eat definitely affects how we feel, but it's also true that how we feel affects what we eat. Jane Haines describes this well. Jane has suffered from Premenstrual Dysphoric Disorder (PMDD) – a more severe form of premenstrual syndrome that can cause depression and anxiety – and she told me:

> 'I don't eat a lot of processed foods as a rule. But I do know that whilst experiencing PMDD symptoms I was way more likely to opt for rubbish food, high fat, high sugar, both as craving and self-punishing, so in that sense it fed the cycle of failure/guilt that very often comes with PMDD. In fact, I would say that eating crap food was one of my three main factors in feelings of failure and guilt and had been since I first experienced PMDD. I don't like the term 'comfort eating' because it was never a comfort; it was always an act of self-loathing, and the food was not healthy, it was the high-fat, high-sugar, zillion-ingredients-on-the-label stuff. Many women on a PMDD forum I am on share similar patterns of behaviour – being health-conscious, but when experiencing symptoms, reaching for processed crap and then spiralling.'

This negative spiral will be familiar to many women, not just those with PMDD. There is something about UPF that makes it the product of choice for women with depression, PMT, PMDD, binge-eating disorder, bulimia and other forms of emotional or disordered eating (see Chapter 5). Part of this is due to the fast, reliable dopamine hit that UPF provides, firing up our brain's reward systems in a similar way to smoking or other addictive behaviours. But it's also possible that this behaviour is connected to another area of our brains impacted by UPF – the hippocampus.

The hippocampus is a relatively small part of the brain, thought to play a role in memory, learning and emotion. It's smaller in people with major depression, and several studies have found that it's impacted by diet. One piece of research found that high UPF intake is associated with a smaller hippocampus, and it would seem that UPF can have a rapid impact on this area of the brain.[48] In a study in 2023, people (predominantly women) who normally ate a healthy diet were asked to eat a high-fat and -sugar diet, including Belgian waffles for breakfast and fast-food takeaways.[49] Within just a week, their learning and memory were affected and, tellingly, they also displayed poorer appetite control. Researchers speculate that the hippocampus is key here: Richard Stevenson, a Professor of Psychology at Macquarie University in Sydney, who led the study, told me: 'The hippocampus seems to be a very vulnerable brain structure. Nobody knows why, but there are several theories swilling around. UPF diets seem to rapidly impair hippocampal function – they do this in humans, rats and mice. Once hippocampal function is disrupted, it then becomes harder to regulate appetite. So you eat more junk food, damage the hippocampus more, and so get into a vicious cycle leading to weight gain and obesity.'

Professor Stevenson directed me to Terry Davidson, Professor of Neuroscience at American University in Washington D.C., who first proposed this 'vicious-cycle model' of obesity. His model proposes that diets high in saturated fats and sugars increase the permeability of the hippocampal blood-brain barrier (BBB), and this allows toxins to enter hippocampal cells. He explained: 'A main function of the hippocampus is to mediate certain memory processes. Our data with rats indicates that the ability to inhibit retrieval of strong memories depends on the hippocampus (termed memory-retrieval inhibition). For example, when one is food-sated, the ability to inhibit retrieval of the memories of food rewards and the pleasures of eating is adaptive.' In other words, the hippocampus stops us from indulging in those 'food fantasies' where we sink our teeth into a juicy cheeseburger or feel the square of chocolate melt in our mouth. Davidson went on to say:

'If a person can't keep those thoughts in check, they are more likely to eat in response to the many food cues that are associated with rewarding foods and eating in the current environment. This eating would occur when food intake is not needed and when one's attention could be better directed toward other activities. Among the most powerful of those environmental cues are the ones that are associated with food high in saturated fats and sugars (very tasty, very rewarding). According to the vicious-cycle account, the more one eats of those foods, the greater the increase in hippocampal pathophysiology (dysfunction), the less able one is to inhibit the memories of those food rewards, the more a person will eat in response to cues associated with those foods when they are food-sated, and on and on. The result is not only increasing hippocampal dysfunction, but also increasing body weight.'

Davidson then slightly blows my mind by explaining that this vicious-cycle model seems to be applicable to systems other than eating. For example, rats who are given cocaine also seem to suffer the same hippocampal-dependent memory problems and inability to stop taking cocaine when sated. And these vicious cycles can be linked: another way to get rats to lose their ability to take it easy on the cocaine, for example, is to keep them on a Western diet. When it comes to depression, Davidson suggests that the same hippocampal impairment may be in play: 'One can argue that a primary symptom of depression is a weakened ability to inhibit negative emotional thoughts and memories. Therefore, based on the vicious-cycle model, diet and other factors that can impair hippocampal function could promote the type of emotional dysregulation that defines depression.' He stresses that this is only speculation. 'However, I do think it is interesting that drugs known as GLP-1 agonists, which are the active agents in the current weight-loss sensations Ozempic and Wegovy, have also been reported to reduce substance abuse and improve hippocampal-dependent cognitive functioning.'

Neither Davidson nor Stevenson has found any clear signs of sex differences in their respective research, but talking to them left me wondering about the predominantly female activity of emotional eating and how this could in turn be impairing the hippocampus, making us more depressed and in the mood for UPF. Food addiction, which almost always means an addiction to UPF, is substantially more common among women, and is frequently co-diagnosed alongside mental health issues, most commonly depression, personality disorder, and schizophrenia.[50] This is potentially yet another vicious cycle: the UPF driving inflammation, disruption to areas of the brain, or other causes of mood disorder – and the mood disorder driving over-consumption of UPF.

Depression and mental health issues are not the only potential negative UPF loop. Insomnia affects 40 per cent more women than men.[51] Having experienced extreme sleep deprivation as a mum of three very wakeful babies, I know first-hand how severe tiredness can fuel unhealthy eating. Cakes and biscuits or a salty, fatty UPF pizza from the freezer can really appeal when you're dead on your feet. But scientists now believe that UPF can actually cause chronic insomnia, both because of the possible impact of UPF on hormones and the microbiome, and because of the deficiency of sleep-promoting nutrients a UPF diet can cause.[52] I can certainly imagine this being yet another vicious cycle – neither preparing nor eating healthy food has much appeal when you're completely exhausted. And the loop continues when you consider that around three-quarters of people with depression have sleep problems,[53] and people with insomnia are around ten times more likely to have depression.[54]

And then there's stress, which also impacts women in much higher numbers than men, and can also propel us towards UPF consumption. Research in mice has found that chronic stress can effectively shut down a part of the brain known as the lateral habenula, not only causing the mice to overeat, with no cut-off point in the positive feelings they gain from indulgence, but also creating a preference for sugary food and drinks: long-term stress drives 'comfort eating', said the researchers, in mice at least.[55] Life circumstances such as poverty, divorce, bereavement or illness can also not only cause stress but lead to depression and unhealthy eating, again adding to this network of overlapping cycles.

The impact of UPF on women's mental health needs much more attention and research. The vicious cycles involved can be complex and interconnected: obesity, poor mental health, disordered eating, low energy, reduced physical activity, low self-esteem, adverse childhood experiences, low libido, poor sleep, poverty, relationship difficulties, and more – all interacting and offering themselves as both cause and effect. If you are reading this, you may yourself be experiencing some or many of these spirals and wondering how you can break free. Perhaps it's worth remembering that, just as small steps and micro-choices can take you into vicious cycles, even small changes may just as easily launch new 'virtuous cycles'. Just one apple a day could give your gut microbes that little bit of extra fibre they need to produce a few more serotonin-enhancing compounds; replacing Diet Coke with water or a cup of tea could give your body a break from artificial sweeteners; taking an omega-3 supplement or starting a weekly fish supper could reduce inflammation. And feeling that tiny bit better could nudge you towards making more positive changes, just as feeling worse can so easily nudge you towards UPF. By creating vicious cycles, you've proven the method works, now you just need to switch it to your advantage – and kick start a few virtuous ones, which will undoubtedly then spiral and grow into patterns you have no desire to break free from.

9.

Ageing like fine cheese

UPF in the second half of life

It was really because of my own 'menopause journey' (as some poetically call it) that I found myself writing this book. As I began to experience menopause 'symptoms' (hmm, funny to have 'symptoms' on a 'journey'?!) in my mid- to late forties, I started to research my options. I looked at some of the standard advice and a few of the popular books and influencers. I read a lot about HRT and I wasn't ruling it out, but as someone who has always been drawn to the more 'natural' path, I was curious about the alternatives. Just as I was starting to feel a little bit like this might be one situation in life where there really *weren't* any alternatives – it was either 'suffer' or 'medicate' – I had a moment of curiosity and did an online search, and it was a game-changer. Here's what I typed into the search box:

How do women experience menopause in other cultures?

What I read really shocked me – menopause symptoms are not universal. For example, until recently there was apparently no word for 'hot flush' in Japanese, so rare is this experience for Japanese women.[1] Other countries also report fewer vasomotor symptoms (that's the overall 'hotting up') than women in the West, with only 5 per cent of Indonesian women reporting hot flushes. (Although some report different symptoms instead, with body and joint pain reported as the predominant issue in many Asian countries.[2]) And it's not just Asia – the First Nations women in Canada, for example, were said by researchers not to 'conceptually link' menopause to 'symptoms typical of menopause from a medical perspective' and explained that they did not have a word for 'menopause'.[3] Mayan women from Yucatán in Mexico reported no symptoms of menopause at all,[4] and the women of the Hadza in Tanzania, one of the world's last remaining hunter-gatherer populations, reported only one: vaginal dryness.[5] The Hadza also have no word for menopause.

It seems to be the case that women in the USA, Canada, Australia and the UK all have a markedly worse experience than women in other parts of the world,[6] to the point that many of us dread this phase of life – but why? Some researchers point to cultural values: in the West, women tend to feel that youth, beauty and fertility signify worth, and therefore menopause is to be feared as an ending, a loss, a negative transition. Other countries frame things differently – in Japan, menopause is called *konenki*, which translates as 'time of renewal and regeneration'; in China, it is known as *second spring*; in the Māori language, a woman becomes *ruahine*, which signifies 'second woman' and also 'woman of importance' or 'wise woman'. When menopause is seen as a kind of upgrade or promotion, women tend to feel more positively towards it and therefore less likely to feel they are 'suffering', even at a physical level, it seems.

A gut-menopause connection?

The reading I did after that quick online search changed everything. It encouraged me to consider that not every woman has the typical British menopause that I was expecting. And it got me thinking more critically about what I was eating and the Western diet. I wondered if my own experience of perimenopause could potentially be shaped by both my mindset and my food, and I began to experiment.

If you're interested in the secret to a long and healthy life, you've probably already read about women in Japan, and particularly in Okinawa, which has the highest ratio of centenarians and supercentenarians (people who live to 110) in the world, almost all of whom are women. What they eat in Okinawa is completely different from the Standard American Diet – they really do follow food writer Michael Pollan's famous advice: 'Eat food, not too much, mostly plants.' Only about 2 per cent of their plate is fish or meat, the rest is vegetables, legumes, rice, and a lot of sweet potatoes. They also eat foods made with soy, like tofu and miso,[7] and it's this that researchers speculate could be the source of their easier menopause, because soy contains something called phytoestrogens, compounds that have a very similar structure to oestrogen.[8] It's oestrogen that drops in perimenopause, and it's this drop that's responsible for the various 'symptoms'. I'm not such a fan of tofu, but another quick search told me that there were other foods that had similar properties. Flax seeds, for example, contain a phytoestrogen called lignan, and walnuts, which I had coincidentally developed a massive craving for in perimenopause, are another source.

I started to consciously eat more foods high in phytoestrogen, in particular at breakfast, where I ditched the UPF cereal I'd had every morning for most of my life and loaded up instead on flax seeds, nuts and berries. Sometimes I had them with natural yoghurt, another source of phytoestrogen, and sometimes with oats – which give the microbiome a good dose of the fibre it needs to process the phytoestrogens. I'm only a sample of one, but within a week or two I started to feel a lot better. There's some research into phytoestrogens in perimenopause that seems to back me up, too, suggesting they may reduce hot flushes and improve bone density, without any harmful effects.[9]

We're not here to talk about my menopause, but in case it's helpful, I will just add that I've also experimented with weight training, which I've found really helpful. Above all, I've tried to pay attention to my feelings and be really kind to myself, in particular by consistently challenging my own negative ideas, given to me by my culture, about my relevance – or lack of it – as I age. I have struggled at times, and think I could have made things even better for myself if I'd cut out alcohol, which always seemed to coincide with my sleepless nights. But hurrah, I'm out the other side of menopause now, and I have not taken HRT. This doesn't mean that I never will, and it's not a judgement on anyone who does because

I know many women who have found HRT a lifeline. But coming at it from a different angle has definitely worked for me, and I really do feel a lot stronger and healthier – in body and mind – than ever before. That one flash of thought about women in other parts of the world prompted me to ask a simple but essential question: 'does it have to be this way?' And the answer seemed to be, no, it doesn't: instead of deciding you're on the scrap heap, you can think about yourself as being renewed and promoted to Wise Woman, and that might help; and instead of eating Special K, you can have a big bowl of phytoestrogens, and that might help. You can do these things alongside HRT, too – it's not an either/or situation. And if you've come this far in this book it won't be a surprise for you to discover that there's something else that's consistently different in every single culture where menopause is less of a problem to be fixed – they don't eat UPF.

Follow the money

The sidelining of women's health issues and the sidelining of older women makes for a menopause Venn diagram so overlapping it's basically a circle. For a long time, menopause received barely any focus from either science or culture, and it's only in recent years that this has started to change. Menopause has become a trending topic – and a lucrative market, with business positively booming in everything from new forms of HRT to ridiculous products like UPF 'Menopause chocolate'. The focus often seems to be on capitalizing on women's suffering rather than alleviating it. One American headline from 2024 sums it up: 'This overlooked corner of women's health could be a $350 billion market opportunity.'[10] It's not surprising, then, that the simple and much less lucrative solution of diet often doesn't get a look-in, and that research into the specific impact of UPF on menopause is still fairly scarce. Joyce Harper, menopause expert and Professor of Reproductive Science at University College London, agrees:

> 'The impact of diet and lifestyle on menopause is totally under-discussed, both at grass-roots level in the consulting room and at the level of policy, research and public information. HRT has a place but should be seen as just one tool in the menopause toolkit, rather than the ultimate solution to everything. If a woman does not listen to her body at this time, or ideally in the years leading up to menopause, then even HRT may not be able to help as much as it should. But this is not generally the message that women are getting.'

The research that has been done, however, is pretty clear: avoiding UPF and eating a Mediterranean-style diet of mostly plants instead *will* have an impact on your menopause experience, and even on the effectiveness of HRT, should you choose to use it. One study in 2022 looked at the effect of food on women's menopause symptoms according to the degree of processing.[11] They found that the highest level of UPF consumption was associated with more intense vasomotor symptoms and, quite specifically, that those drinking sugar-sweetened drinks and eating sausages were most likely to suffer physical symptoms and have issues with their memory and concentration. Those in the study eating less UPF and more vegetables, on the other hand, reported lower menopause symptom intensity and a better quality of life.

Other studies confirm this relationship between a healthy diet, high in fibrous fruit and vegetables, and a reduction in menopause symptoms, with many also showing that UPF, along with saturated fats and sugars, make women feel worse.[12] In 2013 researchers in Australia found that a high-fat and -sugar diet increased the risks of hot flushes, whilst eating a Mediterranean-style diet meant less of such symptoms.[13] Another study that followed over 17,000 post-menopausal women in the USA showed a decrease in vasomotor symptoms in those who ate five servings of fruit and vegetables a day and six servings of whole grains – but found that the improvements were strongest in those women who also lost weight as part of the regimen.[14] And in 2019 another piece of research had similar findings: a diet high in fruits and vegetables reduces menopause symptoms, whilst a diet high in fat, sweets, snacks and desserts increased not just hot flushes but all symptoms.[15] More recently, a large-scale study from personalized nutrition company ZOE has found that menopausal women who consume plenty of whole-plant foods are 30 per cent less likely to report hot flushes and sleep disturbances.[16] Overall, the ZOE data show that diet could have the biggest influence on the menopause experience – with a massive 34 per cent reduction in overall symptoms in those women following a healthy diet.[17] But there's something else that also has a big impact: BMI (body mass index).

Menobelly

What a word that is, and yes, I have one. Having been one of those people who had always been able to eat and drink what I liked and remain a size 10 all my life, perimenopause came along and wiped that smug smile off my face. I got a double dose, as well, because my 'peri' phase coincided with the Covid lockdowns, in other words a couple of years of sitting around the house, begging my children to do online maths, and mainlining the wine and cheese each night in the absence of anything better to do. After a while of wondering whether there was something wrong with my washing machine, I realized that no, my knickers were not shrinking: I was expanding. Once the penny dropped, I began to try every method under the sun to shift those pandemic pounds, but to no avail. Whereas in my twenties and thirties a week or so of self-restraint would have been enough to lose a few kilograms, suddenly, mid-forties, the scales just wouldn't budge. I am not obese, but this experience has taught me a lot about how weight-loss advice is very often ignorant of the perimenopausal demographic, and of women's individual efforts and struggles. I don't have any miracle solutions to offer women in my position, but what I would say is this: if you're reading this and have not yet reached perimenopause, now is a very good time to start looking after yourself and listening to your body, because your menopausal self really will thank you later.

Mid-life may also be the tipping-point we need to overhaul our health, resulting in a new beginning. Helen Duncan, from Sheffield, had spent a lifetime struggling with her weight, but it was when she turned fifty that this became more serious.

'I'd always had a BMI at the top end, around 25,' she told me. 'But after fifty this began to increase and I found myself two-and-a-half stone overweight with a BMI of 30. The thought of another diet filled me with dread. I was always constantly thinking about food and craving food. I know now that it wasn't "food" that I was craving, but UPF.' Helen feels that this addiction started as a child, with the high-sugar, highly refined baby biscuits known as Farley's Rusks. 'My UPF addiction went from there, and became mainly about sweet, fatty foods like cakes and chocolate. But whereas losing weight had previously required a lot of willpower, once I learned about UPF, what it contains and how it is made, this took willpower out of the equation. I no longer see it as food, and instead it repulses me. If you offered me a Krispy Kreme doughnut now, I would look at you with horror.' Helen lost three stone in six months and says she feels better not only physically but mentally because she has broken free from what she sees as a toxic dieting culture. 'I no longer think about food obsessively,' she says. 'Of course I had to completely overhaul my way of eating, but it wasn't difficult because deciding not to eat UPF makes clear the food choices that you have to make. People say that it's difficult and that supermarkets are a minefield. Actually, it's totally easy. Most things that are pre-made and in packets are basically UPF. That leaves you with whole natural foods that need to be cooked from scratch. When my friend found out that I was no longer going to be eating my favourite brand of chocolate she exclaimed that there had to be some joy in life. I explained to her that the pain over the last fifty years of constant yo-yo dieting caused by sugar and UPF far outweighed any joy to be had from eating it. Besides that, I no longer consider it, or any UPF, to be food, so I don't miss it.'

Whilst for Helen, extreme weight gain was something she felt she needed to address, some change in the way our body distributes fat is normal in perimenopause, according to naturopathic doctor and women's hormone expert Lara Briden. She told me: 'A redistribution of fat from the bum to the belly is common. It occurs because we become relatively low in oestrogen, which would normally promote bum fat, and relatively high in testosterone, which – in women – promotes belly fat. Some degree of menopausal thickening around the waist is probably inevitable and not something to worry about too much.' Larger amounts of belly fat could, however, be a sign of insulin resistance or pre-diabetes, says Briden, and this is far more common for modern women in menopause than it was even a couple of generations ago. 'Put it this way,' she explains, 'the menopause transition slightly increases the risk for insulin resistance. For previous generations, that might not have been a problem because their overall risk was low. Now – thanks to the modern food supply and environment – everyone is already at high risk of insulin resistance, so the slightly higher risk with menopause can be enough to push many women into metabolic dysfunction.'

Insulin resistance

Insulin resistance happens when cells in your muscles, fat and liver don't respond well to insulin and can't easily take up glucose from your blood. As a result, your pancreas keeps producing more and more insulin in an attempt to regulate your blood sugar, typically leading to Type 2 diabetes, obesity, non-alcoholic fatty liver disease and cardiovascular disease, and it is also associated with polycystic ovary syndrome (PCOS). UPF is known to play a significant role in every single one of these health issues, with multiple studies linking its consumption to Type 2 diabetes.[18] Some suggest this is due to UPF's high sugar, salt, fat and energy content, coupled with low fibre; other research has investigated the common UPF additive carrageenan and found an association with insulin resistance,[19] and has raised concerns over other additives, such as MSG and sweeteners, as factors in obesity and diabetes.[20] You don't have to be obese to develop insulin resistance or Type 2 diabetes, but your risk increases with your waist circumference. UPF, definitively and without doubt a key driver of disease and obesity, is not doing your menopausal body – future or present – a single favour.[21]

A recent study in the USA has suggested that women living with obesity may not only have worse symptoms of menopause but may also find their HRT less effective, which the study authors speculate may be because of the impact of BMI on drug metabolism.[22] The ZOE research also found that high BMI has a significant impact on the likelihood of suffering with menopausal symptoms, including hot flushes, dry skin, low libido and mood changes. In their research, mood changes were found in about 60 per cent of women with a healthy weight, compared to around 70 per cent of women living with severe obesity. When it came to the numbers suffering hot flushes, these figures were 54 per cent for those with a healthy weight, and 66 per cent for those with severe obesity. And their study also suggests that those women who eat a healthy diet will have fewer menopause symptoms, even if they have a high BMI, and regardless of whether or not they choose to use HRT.[23]

Menopause is a wake-up call for our health. Perhaps this is why our body stubbornly refuses to simply 'lose weight' on the old 'input-output' system we're used to. This time it wants something more. It wants radical self-care. The stress hormone, cortisol, works in balance with oestrogen: when cortisol goes up, oestrogen goes down.[24] Stress and sleep deprivation (both huge factors for me in the pandemic) can also impact our metabolism at this time of life and lead to unhealthy food and drink choices. As our oestrogen drops, changing where our bodies distribute fat, our body shape will probably change to some extent. Part of the work of menopause is self-love for and self-acceptance of both this changing body and a different face in the mirror. But taking care of ourselves through practices like yoga, meditation, early nights, reduced alcohol, journalling, therapy, strength training and a better diet are also more important than ever. It's the perfect time to quit or reduce UPF and replace it with food that really nourishes you. HRT can also be helpful, so use it if you need it, but if you are not practising radical self-care, then it's possible that even HRT won't have the impact you are hoping for. I was recently asked for menopause advice by a person I know who is a heavy drinker. She had tried various forms of HRT, but still felt so awful that she had to take time off work. Why was menopause hitting her so hard? The answer was obvious, but like all of us at times, she was hoping for a solution that didn't involve her having to change.

Menopause is literally called The Change. It demands we do things differently and its messages are loud and clear. If we don't want to hear them, unfortunately we can expect a rougher ride.

Size isn't everything

Much dietary advice for perimenopausal women revolves around the *size* of their plates rather than what is actually *on* their plates. We need to rethink this completely.

Karen Newby is a nutritionist and author of *The Natural Menopause Method*, and she agrees that the current lack of focus on what to eat for a better menopause is frustrating: 'There is so little discussion on the role of nutrition and how it can help menopausal symptoms and at the same time future-proof your health. It's a total win-win! But instead, my whole area of study often gets brushed aside as just "eat a balanced diet" – well, what does a balanced diet even mean? We need a *therapeutic* diet at menopause.' This focus away from nutrition and onto 'weight loss' sets women up to fail, she argues, because of the underlying hormonal reasons for weight gain. 'And this is where the ultra-processed food market swoops in,' she notes. 'Heavily marketed to women with slogans like "go-ahead" and calorie-led products, which are all full of non-food. Instead of anchoring our hunger, they create cravings for more. This then creates a feeling of guilt around food. Menopause is hard enough, let alone feeling guilty about what we're eating or feeling like we're going without.'

So a plate overflowing with fresh, home-cooked whole food and plants will nurture us through this phase of life far better than a 'small plate' of UPF. Our menopausal bodies, with their lowered oestrogen, are more susceptible to inflammation than our younger selves and can also have more extreme blood sugar responses or 'spikes' – both risk factors for chronic disease like Type 2 diabetes, heart disease and obesity. Protein is also really important at this time when we tend to lose muscle mass, and will also help us keep our blood sugar on an even keel. So it's not so much about eating LESS, with the exception of:

- less sugary foods, especially factory-made cakes, biscuits and desserts;
- quit or reduce soda/fizzy drinks, fruit juice, smoothies and alcohol;
- quit or reduce UPF.

And in their place, the focus needs to be on eating MORE, particularly of certain types of food:

- more oily fish (omega-3 = anti-inflammatory);
- more plants (prebiotics, polyphenols, micronutrients, fibre);
- more whole grains (rice, quinoa, oats, barley, rye, corn);
- more legumes (lentils, peas, beans);
- more phytoestrogens (soya (tofu, tempeh, edamame), flax seed, linseed, nuts, garlic);
- more protein (from legumes, meat, fish, nuts, seeds, eggs, tofu);
- more fermented foods (probiotics).

Gutsy old women

Mid-life is also the perfect time to give some love and care to your microbiome, which, just like menopausal women themselves, goes through a time of upheaval and change. Our gut microbes play a key role in regulating our metabolism, and the oestrobolome (see Chapter 6) is in charge of regulating our circulating oestrogen. At menopause, it seems like our microbial composition changes and can become less diverse, which potentially brings health risks. Health in old age is reflected not just in diversity of gut microbes, but in an ever-increasing uniqueness in their composition – just as we become less interested in conforming as we grow older, so, it seems, do our resident bacteria.[25] One study has found that our colony of gut microbes after menopause also becomes more similar to those found in men,[26] whilst other research has suggested that taking HRT mitigates some of these microbial changes,[27] although this is not yet clear.[28]

So much more research is needed in this area that scientists have described it as 'an unexplored new frontier in peri- and post-menopausal health'.[29] The implications for women in the second half of their lives are vast, and there are many unanswered questions. How does the microbiome influence our menopause experience? In what way does HRT help or hinder our microbes, and vice versa? How much are mental health issues like depression in middle age related to our gut? And what role do our changing menopausal microbes play in disease in later life? Until we know more, the same advice about supporting the health of your gut microbes at any stage of life applies: eat more fibre from plants (prebiotics), more live and fermented foods (probiotics), and avoid UPF, which not only doesn't have the fibre your microbes crave but may also disrupt their functioning at this critical time.

Gallstones: messages from within

One issue with gut health that affects people in mid-life and beyond is gallstones. These are tiny crystals that develop inside the gallbladder, which is the part of the digestive system that stores bile (that greenish-yellow liquid you might have seen when vomiting) and helps digest fats. It's estimated that between 5 per cent and 25 per cent of people have gallstones – some without knowing – and they are as much as three times more common in women than men. Long thought to be a part of the body that, like the appendix, we can manage without, the gallbladder is removed by a procedure known as a cholecystectomy. More than 60,000 such procedures are performed each year in the UK,[30] on a demographic apparently described by doctors as 'female, fair, fat, fertile and forty'.

Lynne Pratt developed gallbladder issues at 62 and believes it was directly related to her consumption of UPF. 'I was an ice-cream addict,' she told me. 'I loved sausages. I loved chocolate. I loved desserts with cream. I ate "bought" cakes and biscuits. I ate these in quantity and I was very overweight.' While she was waiting for her gallbladder removal surgery to be scheduled, Lynne changed her diet – for the most part because any highly processed or fatty food caused her pain. 'By the time I got my op, I was eating rice crackers, oatcakes, boiled eggs and boiled vegetables. Plain pasta was an adventure. I lost a lot of weight, nearly six stone. In spite of my pain and health issues, I was in many ways healthier. I could walk further, swim further and I had more energy. With the help of my GP, I continued to change my diet.' After the surgery, Lynne put some weight back on but says she is no longer overweight. 'I feel much better about walking, swimming, and exercising in general. I have energy and enthusiasm. I think this is down to a mixture of cutting out highly processed food and losing sufficient weight to live better.'

Lynne's story is supported by the evidence. Combined analysis of three large studies, published in July 2024, showed that the more UPF consumed, the greater the risk of gallstones, and pointed the finger in particular at drinks, both sugar-sweetened and artificially sweetened.[31] Worryingly, although gallstones have traditionally been an issue for mid-life and beyond, experts say more and more younger women are presenting with them, it's thought due to obesity and poor diet.[32] In mild cases, it may be possible to manage gallbladder issues through diet, rather than surgery. Kate Horton was 44 years old when she started experiencing pain and was offered a cholecystectomy. 'But I explained to my doctor – it's not that I can't eat fruit and vegetables, it's that I can't eat McDonald's, shop-bought cakes and biscuits, crisps, fish and chips, and all these things that are bad for me. These were the foods that caused pain. And something didn't feel right to me about undergoing an anaesthetic, having an organ removed, it felt like a quick fix when actually I should have been listening to my body.' Her surgeon eventually agreed with her analysis that it was her diet that was the problem rather than her gallbladder, and instead of accepting surgery, she now avoids all UPF, has regular colonic hydrotherapy and takes daily Milk Thistle, long used as a herbal remedy for liver, kidney and gallbladder issues. Whilst this may not be the right path for everyone – and anyone with gallstones should consult their doctor – Kate feels that dietary changes worked in her case. 'On the one rare occasion I did eat UPF – a bacon and pancake breakfast, a hot dog and a cupcake – I immediately got a gallbladder attack. My body rejected it, none of that was good for me. But without my gallbladder, how would I have known how much my body was rejecting that food? It occurred to me then how many people – and mainly women – were just having this organ, and quite possibly its warning signals, taken away, silenced.'

Ultra-processed skeletons

Another concern of older women is osteoporosis – when bones get weaker and break more easily. If you are at risk, for example if you have a family history of osteoporosis or have already had fractures, you may be referred for a DEXA scan in your fifties. Women are more at risk of osteoporosis, it's thought due to the impact of the drop in oestrogen post-menopause, which can lead to a decrease in bone density. Diet has long been promoted as key to osteoporosis prevention, with emphasis on calcium intake and Vitamin D, and a number of studies have found a link between UPF consumption and bone density, particularly on the growing skeleton. One piece of research fed young rats a UPF diet high in fat and sugar and found that they suffered from growth retardation and that their bone mineral density decreased significantly, resulting in bones with a 'sieve-like' appearance and a high risk of fracture.[33] Another fed groups of young female mice different diets and found that the UPF group had impaired bone quality due to high-fat deposits in their bone marrow, which scientists speculate happened as a result of their altered gut microbiomes.[34] Another interesting study, this time in humans, found that children who lived near fast-food outlets, as opposed to near community stores, had significantly lower bone mineral density by the age of four.[35] Other studies have found that regular fizzy drinks are associated with osteoporosis[36] and that cola, in particular, is linked with low bone density in older women.[37] This information is something to bear in mind if you play a role in feeding your own or other people's kids – but does it mean that it's too late for your bones if you've been drinking Coke or had a UPF diet most of your life? Kirsty Carne, Senior Osteoporosis Specialist Nurse at the Royal Osteoporosis Society, says that it's not too late:

> 'Our bones keep renewing themselves throughout life, so it's never too late to make changes that can help keep your bones healthy. These include eating a balanced diet containing a wide range of different foods from the four main groups (fruit and vegetables, carbohydrates, dairy and dairy alternatives, and proteins) and ensuring that you consume enough calcium to give your bones their strength. Lifestyle changes, such as being active, reducing alcohol intake and stopping smoking, also play an important role in maintaining good bone health. Safe exposure to sunlight is

essential for receiving enough Vitamin D, which helps your body to absorb calcium, so if you live in a part of the world with darker winter months, you should consider taking a daily supplement of 10mg (400 units) of Vitamin D.'

When it comes to protecting our bones as we age, it seems we can definitely take a proactive approach.

Thinking ahead

Just as when we are in our thirties we often avoid thinking about our menopausal selves, when we are in mid-life we tend to avoid thinking about ourselves entering old age. But the seeds of change we sow today have the potential to reap benefits tomorrow, and quitting UPF now might well protect us from what is many people's greatest fear in their later years: dementia.

Women have all the more reason to be concerned about dementia. We are twice as likely as men to get the most common form of it – Alzheimer's disease – and dementia is the leading cause of death for women, remaining in this top spot even during the Covid pandemic. Women over the age of 60 years are twice as likely to develop Alzheimer's during the rest of their lifetime as they are to get breast cancer. In the USA, there are five million Americans with Alzheimer's, and two-thirds of them are women;[38] in the UK, 982,000 people are living with dementia,[39] and again, two-thirds are women.[40] And dementia doesn't just upturn the lives of those diagnosed: 15 million Americans are currently providing care and support for those suffering, and two-thirds of these carers are women.

At the risk of sounding like a stuck record, it probably won't surprise you to know that this, like every other area of women's health, is hugely under-researched. Analysis from Alzheimer's Research UK has even found that, whilst the majority of dementia researchers are female, they are less likely to be awarded research grants and less likely to become senior academics than their male counterparts.[41] Against this backdrop we don't even yet know why twice as many people with Alzheimer's are female – it used to be thought that it was simply because women tend to live slightly longer, but now scientists are exploring the impact of declining oestrogen and drawing connections with the ways in which menopause impacts the brain, such as brain fog and insomnia. However, it is important to be clear that the 'brain fog' of menopause is not the same as dementia or cognitive decline, and that although it can cause women to worry that they will never be the same again, it's a temporary state – except in very rare cases where it is an early sign of dementia. Where menopausal brain fog may cause us to forget things or feel we cannot quite think straight (for example, where are my car keys?), dementia impacts our ability to function in our daily life (for example, being lost in a familiar place).

Lisa Mosconi, neuroscientist and author of *The XX Brain*, emphasizes the role of a 'Mediterranean diet' in both menopausal health and Alzheimer's prevention, in particular the consumption of foods rich in phytoestrogens, such as flax and sesame seed, soy beans, legumes, and a number of fruits and vegetables.[42] 'Exercise is the first line of attack,' she says.[43] 'Diet is the second – so up your plant game.' A study in Brazil in 2023 directly linked the consumption of UPF to cognitive decline: from an analysis of over 10,000 people in their fifties over a period of eight years, researchers found that those who consumed the highest amount of UPF had a 28 per cent faster decline in cognitive scores, including memory, verbal fluency and the ability to plan and execute goals, compared to those with a lower consumption of UPF.[44] The study also found this association was stronger in older adults, suggesting that it's never too late to make changes to what you eat, but that the sooner you do so, the more you may lower your risk for cognitive decline.

As noted above, cognitive decline is not the same as dementia, although it can be an early sign of the disease. But another study, published in the journal *Neurology* in 2022, was more specific about the link between UPF consumption and dementia itself.[45] Researchers looked at data from over 70,000 people, in a database called the UK Biobank, over a ten-year period and examined their diets and whether or not they went on to develop forms of dementia, including Alzheimer's. They found a clear relationship between high consumption of UPF and dementia risk and, similarly, that reducing UPF reduced that risk: replacing 10 per cent of UPF in your diet with an equivalent amount of unprocessed or minimally processed food could lower your dementia risk by around 19 per cent. Why would this be?

At the moment, experts still don't have clear answers. We know that a diet high in UPF increases the risk of cerebrovascular disease[46] – a term for conditions that affect blood flow to the brain. We also know that high UPF is associated with a smaller hippocampus (see page 180), the part of the brain associated with learning and memory. The authors of the study in *Neurology* also speculate that there could be a connection with high-salt consumption, or with the plastic packaging of UPF. And other research points to the microbiome: scientists are now discovering that the brain itself has a microbiome, and that certain species of bacteria are only present in the brains of people with Alzheimer's – with the implied potential that some dementias could eventually be reversible.[47] Researchers have also found connections between dementia and the oral microbiome, and suggest both good oral hygiene and diet can be factors in preventing dysbiosis (microbiome imbalance).[48] The brain bacteria of Alzheimer's patients is said to be 'inflammation promoting',[49] and other research into dementia suggests a link with the inflammatory nature of the Western diet caused by disruption to our gut microbes.[50] And if old age sounds too far off to worry about, it's worth remembering that younger people get dementia too: Dementia UK estimates that around 7.5 per cent of people living with dementia in the UK were diagnosed between the ages of 30 and 64 years.[51] Again, a disproportionate amount of these people living with young onset dementia will be female.

Strong and vintage

It has been well established that a healthy diet has a positive impact on longevity,[52] and conversely there is plenty of evidence linking UPF to cancer, heart disease and other causes of death.[53] A large study of Italian adults in November 2024, in which scientists looked at 36 different markers in the participants' blood, showed that a diet rich in UPF was associated with the acceleration of biological ageing.[54] In the world's 'Blue Zones' – the areas of the world said to have the longest-living populations[55] – you won't find anyone eating Pringles. In Okinawa, the Blue Zone in Japan where, you'll recall, they don't have a word for 'hot flush' (page 185–186), they eat a largely plant-based diet. In another Blue Zone, Ikaria in Greece, where they are almost entirely free of dementia and where one in three lives to their nineties, they eat a Mediterranean diet, just as they do in another Blue Zone, the Italian island of Sardinia. And in Nicoya, Costa Rica, they eat the 'three sisters' – squash, beans and corn – and put their extremely strong bones in old age down to the high levels of calcium in their drinking water. We all want to live longer, but for many of us this actually means 'live better' – we want to be fit and healthy in old age rather than simply being chair-bound and racking up the birthdays. There are more factors than diet to achieving this: genes, having a sense of purpose, being active, and feeling supported by community are all said to help us stay healthy into old age. But changing our relationship with food could bring us some of those elements, too, as we take charge of our own or our loved ones' health, and bring back the human connection that comes when we take time to sit round a table together.

As we age, we may also want to keep looking as young as we can. In a book for women and about women, this is a complex topic to broach – if we are past about 40 years of age, we are well used to the constant pressure not to 'look our age' but rather to devote hours of our time and plenty of our hard-earned cash in the effort to maintain a false illusion of youth – a pressure to which men are not subjected. When I was thinking about the title for this chapter, I came across the delightful maxim: 'Men age like fine wine, women age like milk.' There is forever a double standard in the expectations our culture sets for us in terms of how we look, praising older men for looking 'distinguished' with 'salt-and-pepper hair', whilst older women, in particular the ones who dare to defy convention by 'not bothering', are subjected to the most extraordinary misogyny centred entirely on their personal appearance: like milk, we women in our second half of life are sour and past our best; we have gone bad.

In spite of this, I feel compelled to tell you that you have structures called telomeres at the end of your chromosomes that protect them, rather like shoelace tips protect the shoelace. Over time, your telomeres shorten, and this shortening is thought to be one of the factors that causes cells to age. It won't surprise you to hear that smoking, drinking, obesity and other lifestyle factors can shorten your telomeres, but so too can UPF. Research in Spain in 2020 found that the likelihood of having shortened telomeres increased dramatically with the number of servings, with those in the high UPF consumption group – having three or more a day – being 82 per cent more likely to have shortened telomeres.[56] And if you're truly not fussed about looking older than your years, remember that having shortened telomeres also has implications for your health and lifespan.

Regarding the ageing like milk thing, it has been pointed out that aged milk is, in fact, cheese. As I embrace mid-life, I can't think of anything I'd like to be compared to more than a perfectly aged Parmigiano: firm, salty, complex, rich, sharp and bold.

10.

A delicious tub of face cream

The disturbing overlaps of UPF and cosmetics

When I've told people I'm writing this book, they have often wondered aloud if it's difficult to give up these food items we all know and love. But my own experience has been that, once I began to realize that my luxury snack was a close cousin to my night cream, my appetite for UPF waned rapidly. If you think about the words that some people have used in their attempts to define UPF – 'concoctions', 'confections of confections', 'formulations', 'substances', 'ultra-processed products' – you begin to see that the same terms could be applied to many of the items in our wash bag or make-up set. Aromatic chemical concoctions – I don't mind so much the idea of putting such things on my hair, but I'd really rather not eat them; although doing either is probably 'safe' in the sense that it's very unlikely to cause my immediate demise. But in this chapter I want to show you some of the disturbing overlaps between UPF and cosmetics that, even if they don't stop you applying lippy, may well completely put you off that tray of doughnuts that shares some of the same ingredients. Let's start with a story about the way we choose our food, that leads us to a strange world where you can apply pumpkin-spiced eyeshadow whilst sipping wine that tastes like biscuits.

Sensational women

Once upon a time, food would have been something we had an intimate relationship with: sourcing it was key to our survival, as was ensuring its safety. In our modern times we have outsourced these jobs to the point that we rarely think about them, picking up packages from plentifully stocked shelves and ingesting their contents without question. But for much of our human history, the look, feel and smell of a berry, root or pieces of meat was a hugely important aspect of our eating decision-making. And this vital work, which in some cases could have meant life or death, was one that women were – and still are – much better at than men.

For starters, there's colour. You may not consciously think about this, but when you pick out supermarket fruit or veg, you're assessing their ripeness and tastiness with your eyes, before you reach out and make subsequent assessments with your hands, and perhaps your nose. And if you're female, you're able to perceive far more diversity of colour than if you're male. Women are also very rarely colour-blind – only one in 200 women are affected by it, compared to one in twelve men – and it's thought that only women have tetrachromatic vision, which is the ability to see one hundred million colours instead of the usual one million.[1] These superpowers come from the second X chromosome, which compensates if the other has problems discerning colour, providing women with a 'back-up' on colour perception that men, with their XY genes, don't have. There's also a theory that as the 'gatherer' half of the 'hunter-gatherer' duo, women's better sense of colour perception may have evolved as a way of noticing and choosing the best and safest food to eat, whilst men retain a different ability – they are better at tracking and following moving objects in the distance.[2]

We don't know if the 'gatherer' theory is the full picture – and it's almost certain that many women of the past would have been adept at hunting, too – but it may explain why women have been shown in several studies to have a better sense of smell. We have up to 50 per cent more cells in the olfactory region of the brain than men – the area that is the first to receive signals about odour, sent via the nostrils.[3] And as our ability to smell is intricately related to our sense of taste, it's probably not surprising that women excel in this area, too, particularly women of reproductive age, perhaps because of the importance of rejecting unpleasant and potentially toxic food in pregnancy, or perhaps due to the way we bond with our young. Women are twice as likely as men to be 'supertasters', people who have one hundred times more taste buds per square centimetre than average: in neolithic times, this might have meant we made great foragers; nowadays, it apparently predisposes us towards being naturally better at wine-tasting.[4] One wonders if this supersense also makes women more susceptible to the hyperpalatability of UPF, or even connects to our being seven times more likely than men to develop a food addiction?[5]

A close look at the food industry reveals just how UPF brands manipulate our evolutionary abilities to feel confident and safe when choosing our food, using brightly coloured packaging to attract us, co-opting images of nurturing mothers in their advertising, hypnotizing us with repeated phrases such as 'plant-based', displaying tempting images that don't bear much resemblance to the actual product, and even pumping the delicious smells of fresh coffee or just-baked bread into stores to activate both our appetites and our purchasing powers. These tactics particularly target women, superficially because we often hold the household purse strings and also, at a deeper level, tapping into our evolved sensory powers and biological imperatives to make highly attuned choices. The use of aromas in stores is particularly interesting, because they are very often fake – that is to say, in some cases the shop is not actually baking bread, they are simply pumping out artificially made scents. This marketing strategy is used far more in the USA, but it's increasingly being employed in the UK too – the M&M's store in Leicester Square, for example, apparently infuses the air with a chocolate aroma to compensate for the fact that most of its actual products are pre-packed. And investigating where a fake aroma such as this may come from leads you to a very revealing place, where the two industries of food and cosmetics intersect.

Smells delicious!

If you've ever lost your sense of smell, for example through Covid, you'll know this has a corresponding impact on your ability to taste: this is because your tastebuds can only work out the basics, like 'sweet' or 'salty', and it's your nose and olfactory system that then add in more specific information about flavour. What you might not know, however, is that there is a multi-billion-dollar industry that straddles these two human experiences of 'flavour and fragrance'. Huge global companies like Givaudan, Symrise, and International Flavours and Fragrances (IFF) – all part of a market currently worth over $40 billion[6] – specialize in creating flavours: from your tangy cheese crisps to your strawberry snack bar, they make the stuff described on the ingredients as 'flavouring'. Whether listed as 'natural flavouring' or 'artificial flavouring', both are largely the same: a blend of chemicals, sometimes more than a hundred, put together by professional 'flavourists' and added to food to make it smell and taste like the natural item it mimics: think 'buttery' spread, 'smoky' chicken wings, 'cherry' cola, and so on. These same 'flavour and fragrance' giants also make the aroma of your washing powder, shampoo, soap and deodorant, and they make many of the world's leading brands of perfume.[7] They can make your lip balm smell like Dr Pepper or your nail polish smell like Froot Loops breakfast cereal, just as they can make your milkshake taste of banana even when it doesn't contain any, your bacon crisps entirely suitable for vegetarians, and your Christmas bottle of perfume have top notes of a warm ocean breeze. In each case, whilst ingredients may vary, the same basic processes are used: the manipulation of chemicals in a laboratory. As food writer Eric Schlosser puts it, 'The basic science behind the scent of your shaving cream is the same as that governing the flavour of your TV dinner.'[8]

These industry-overlaps sometimes literally encompass entire brands, for example Unilever, which makes items found in both the kitchen and the bathroom cabinet, such as Hellmann's mayonnaise, Knorr stock cubes, Ben & Jerry's ice cream, Sure deodorant, Dove beauty creams, and Lux soap. Procter & Gamble, who make brands like Olay and Pantene, used to make Pringles (until they sold them to Kellogg's). Maybe it's not surprising, then, that as well as having the same science behind their tastes and aromas, some of these items also have ingredients in common: both the food and beauty industries have found ways to make their products last longer, have smoother textures, and look more appealing – and they share them.

Some examples: EDTA (see page 31), which is used in mayonnaise and salad dressing as a chelating agent, is also found in some deodorants, hair conditioners, face creams and cosmetic foundations. Xanthan gum, that bacterial by-product that's used to thicken and emulsify ice creams and salad dressings (and it seems to be in almost everything, I recently found it my 'honey roast' peanuts), is also in my favourite mascara and a top-brand moisturiser. Then there's maltodextrin, an intensely processed white powder made from plant starch, most often corn. It's in your UPF pizza, your instant noodles, and your energy drinks, but it could also be in that stick you use to cover up your eye bags or your shiny new eye-shadow palette. And the bronzer you love might contain potassium sorbate, a synthetically made form of salt that, if you have a supermarket hummus wrap, is probably in both the hummus and the wrap. Everything from your sugary marshmallow bar to your protein shake might contain the gum extracted from seaweed called carrageenan, and so might your toothpaste.

And your meat-free meatballs might be held together with the thickening compound methyl cellulose, which you might also find in your skin exfoliator, or even your wallpaper paste.

Researching these blurred lines between food and cosmetics is incredibly difficult and time-consuming. Search engines, and even AI, don't have much to say – it's a case of literally looking at labels, one at a time, and making notes, trying to find connections. Some additives are banned in the EU but not in the USA – for example, titanium dioxide was banned as a food whitener in Europe in 2022 as a possible carcinogen, but is still used in America in many products from doughnut frosting to salad dressings.[9] And it's allowed in both parts of the world for use in cosmetics like foundation and bronzer, where it's thought to be less easily absorbed by the body and therefore safe. Tracking down 'what's in what' is made even more complex by the fact that some ingredients have multiple names, for example another additive, dimethicone, is also known as dimethylpolysiloxane and as polydimethylsiloxane (PDMS), or by the E number E900. In the face cream Olay and in Dove deodorant it's labelled as dimethicone, in Herbal Essences conditioner it's bis-aminopropyl dimethicone, on Sainsbury's doughnuts it's dimethylpolysiloxane, and on the cooking oil Crisp 'n Dry it appears as di-methyl polysiloxane (E900). It's used as a lube on condoms, where it's listed as 'silicone'. It also seems, as E900, to be added to some 'bag in box' soft drinks syrups used by pubs, for example Diet Pepsi, but it's not listed on the same-brand cans sold in shops.[10] This is presumably because it's an anti-foaming agent and therefore more useful when it's being forced through a soda-stream but, to be honest, I'm guessing. Information on all of the hows, whys and whats is, frankly, so difficult to find that I was left wondering if this was deliberate. After a while you start to wonder whether any of it really matters and if, even though one or two of these ingredients might not be great for your body, nobody might ever be able to work out which ones these are, and even if they did work it out, you still wouldn't be able to understand it all and so maybe it's easier not to worry so much. Maybe this is deliberate too.

Recipes for disaster

Whether or not the struggle to get clear information on ingredients is accidental, it certainly immediately changes the way you look at your food when you do make the effort. But these shared chemicals are by no means the only worrying overlap between our make-up bag and our shopping bag.

For starters, there's the over-consumption. Just as we often buy more food than we need and then send it – and its packaging – to the bin or recycling box, we often participate in the same throwaway culture with make-up and toiletries. The beauty industry produces around 120 billion pieces of packaging each year, and at the moment much of this is not recycled – it's estimated we throw away around 95 per cent of it. Analysis from the environmental group Plastic Soup has found that plastic is also 'the hidden beauty ingredient', with around nine out of ten of the leading brands containing microplastics.[11] Plastic Soup has a free app, 'Beat the Microbead', that you can use to scan your products to see which, if any, microplastics they contain. Their number one offender is dimethicone – that ingredient mentioned previously (see page 217) that's in everything from shampoo to doughnuts – yes, we are eating this stuff as well as putting it on our bodies. Dimethicone, according to Beat the Microbead, is in 20 per cent of products listed on the database and is 'poorly biodegradable, expected to persist in the environment, and expected to be toxic to aquatic organisms'.[12] According to the Environmental Investigation Agency, at least 633 marine species are affected by microplastics in the water.[13] Other environmental concerns overlap with the food industry – for example, palm oil (see page 233) is in around 70 per cent of beauty products, and its production has caused devastation to vital rainforests and their indigenous peoples. Soy, which also has an environmental impact (see page 235), is also used in the cosmetics industry, with derivatives like hydrogenated soybean oil and soybean glycerides being used in cleansers, sunscreen, make-up and more.

PFAS

If you've ever worried about the safety of the non-stick coating on your frying pan, you might be familiar with the term PFAS – which stands for polyfluoroalkyl and perfluoroalkyl substances – a group of synthetic chemicals that came into use after the invention of Teflon in the 1930s. There are many different types of PFAS, and although those thought to be a serious risk to health have now been banned, there are so many yet to be tested, and other new types still being created.

Known as 'forever chemicals', PFAS contain strong bonds that are difficult to break down naturally, meaning they persist in soils and in the water system, finding their way into fish and wildlife and eventually the human body. It's thought that 99 per cent of Americans now have PFAS in their blood,[14] and a test in 2024 of the hair and blood of several UK politicians found that all of them were contaminated by PFAS, including traces of PFOS, a hazardous form of PFAS that was banned fifteen years ago – demonstrating how long these chemicals stick around.[15]

A BBC investigation in January 2023 found that PFAS were still present in major beauty brands being sold in the UK.[16] In the USA, the Modernization of Cosmetics Regulation Act was passed in 2022, requiring the Food & Drug Administration (FDA) to assess the safety of PFAS in cosmetics, but these findings will not be reported until the end of 2025 – meanwhile, PFAS remain.[17] PFAS in our make-up and face creams may be a concern, but it's thought that food packaging – in direct contact with our food – may pose a greater risk. The environmental charity Fidra found PFAS in packaging collected from eight out of nine major UK supermarkets and in 100 per cent of the takeaways that it tested, with significant levels found in items like bakery bags, pizza boxes, and compostable moulded fibre takeaway boxes.[18] Fidra recommended a simple home test called 'beading' to see if PFAS are present: put a small droplet of olive oil on the surface of your packaging; if it soaks in or spreads, it's probably okay, but if it forms a 'bead' shape, it's likely to contain PFAS. It's thought that, along with food, the highest risk for PFAS is our drinking water, but more research is needed into both the harms of PFAS and ways to remove them from the environment. Globally, countries are now beginning to work together to tackle these issues,[19] but in the meantime people are taking steps to limit PFAS exposure by, for example, filtering water, avoiding takeaways or taking their own glass storage containers to restaurants, and seeking out PFAS-free dental floss.

Phthalates

PFAS have also been found to be present in some, but not all, menstrual products: a US-based study in 2022 found PFAS in 48 per cent of period and incontinence pads, in 22 per cent of tampons, and in 65 per cent of period underwear.[20] The chemicals in our menstrual wear have another overlap with the food and cosmetic industry: phthalates. A 2024 review also found that phthalates are present in our tampons and pads at measurable levels,[21] and another study in 2020 had similar findings, with researchers pointing out that the delicate skin of the vulva and vagina more readily absorbs these chemicals.[22] Perhaps unsurprisingly, they have also been found to be present in disposable nappies.[23]

Phthalates, which make plastic soft and flexible, got a mention on pages 158–159 for their role as possible endocrine disruptors, with potential impact on low birth weight and pre-term birth, and on the AGD (anogenital distance) of the developing male foetus. They have also been associated with an increased risk of diabetes in women in mid-life,[24] and although much of the research into phthalates has focused on male reproductive health, there is increasing data to suggest they may impact women in this area too, potentially contributing to reduced fertility[25] and disorders such as PCOS and endometriosis.[26] Like PFAS, phthalates have been found in measurable levels in the human body,[27] and can also cross the placenta and find their way into breast milk.[28] A study in 2024 from the University of Washington Medical School found that pregnant women whose diets were higher in UPF had higher levels of phthalates in their urine, potentially causing 'oxidative stress and an inflammatory cascade within the foetus', according to researchers.[29] Women have greater exposure to phthalates because of our cosmetic use – they are present in many items from nail polish to hair spray – and women of colour are thought to have the highest exposure because of racial and ethnic differences in beauty product use.[30] There are different regulations on the various phthalates depending on where you are in the world and they may not even appear on the label,[31] in particular if they are used in perfume and other 'scented' products that list 'fragrance' or 'flavour' on their ingredients.[32] These words on food, cosmetics and other household labels, such as fabric softener, can represent dozens of chemical ingredients that companies do not currently have to disclose.

BPA

There are other overlapping chemicals in the worlds of food and cosmetics that warrant a mention. BPA – or Bisphenol A – is used to make rigid plastics such as drinks bottles, the packaging for toiletries, and the protective lining of food cans, as well as most cash register receipts. Although it has now been banned from use in baby bottles and beakers, and from being used as an ingredient in cosmetics, it has been shown to enter the body and affect hormones, including those essential to reproduction. It's also been shown to be an endocrine disrupting chemical (EDC), mimicking the structure and function of the hormone oestrogen, and although research is ongoing, current evidence points to adverse impacts on the female reproductive system,[33] with one 2020 paper describing it as 'an emerging threat to female fertility'.[34] Other studies have raised concerns over the possible impact of BPA during pregnancy on the developing foetus, in particular on brain development, with one study showing its particular impact on emotional and behavioural problems in young girls.[35] Although it is not known why this is, researchers speculate the disruption of oestrogen levels may be involved.[36]

One of the authors of that study is Dr Shanna Swan, Professor of Environmental Medicine and Public Health at Mount Sinai School of Medicine in New York City. Her work specializes in prenatal and early childhood stressors and she is the author of *Count Down*, a book that explores the impact of EDCs, including phthalates and BPA, on both male and female fertility and predicts that assisted reproduction will become the norm if we do not address the issue of EDCs.[37] Professor Swan told me:

'The "critical exposure window" for these EDC chemicals is immediately before conception and during pre-natal development. When exposure occurs at this time, it can interfere with the body's natural hormones and affect multiple systems in the body, including reproductive function, metabolism, immune response, and neurodevelopment. Changes caused by pre-natal exposure (unlike those tied to post-natal exposure) are irreversible. Therefore, it is particularly important that couples planning to conceive, and pregnant women, take steps to reduce exposure to these EDCs – chemicals that can affect hormones. These are found in plastic products, personal care products, cleaning and laundry products and more. Food and drink are major sources of exposure.'

I asked Dr Swann if she had any optimism for this situation being turned around. 'Not without a global effort,' she told me. 'The Global Plastics Treaty, now under negotiation, would be a giant leap forward.' And in the meantime? 'Buy organic food, not wrapped in plastic, do not store food in plastic containers, and never microwave food in plastic!'

Parabens

Parabens are added to cosmetics and personal care products as a preservative, and although they are not used in food in the UK, they turn up elsewhere in the world in the form of the E numbers 214, 215, 218 and 219. Searching around to see if I could find their use in the UK, I was surprised to find them listed as an ingredient, as E214 and E218, in the widely used children's paracetamol Calpol. I also found another, 'propylparaben', listed as an ingredient in Femfresh intimate wash; researchers suggest their use in such products could be a cause for concern given the delicacy of skin in this area.[38] Again, they are thought to be endocrine disrupting and able to mimic the hormone oestrogen. The charity Breast Cancer UK suggests that parabens and other endocrine disruptors could have a role in breast cancer, although there is still not enough evidence to be sure about this, and another cancer charity, Cancer Research UK, states that parabens are not a cancer risk.[39] Breast Cancer UK points out 'the cocktail effect' – we are all exposed to several of these chemicals, via cosmetics, and packaging and food, on a daily basis and it's difficult to know what the risk of one person's particular 'cocktail' might be, even if we have evidence about individual ingredients.[40]

This concept of the 'cocktail effect' certainly resonates when you consider all of the different ways in which our current food, cosmetics, menstrual products and packaging may be impacting upon us – it's mind-boggling and somewhat overwhelming. Just as we have done with UPF, in our quest for convenience and profits we have completely sidelined human health and our impact on nature and future generations. And just as with UPF, it might be time to question whether big corporations and legislators have our best interests at heart. Helen Lynn, health advisor and Environmenstrual Campaign Manager at the Women's Environmental Network (Wen), a UK charity that focuses on gender, health, equality and environmental justice, suggests that the time is up for the current lack of transparency: 'Unless we have the information, we cannot call for change, we cannot choose wisely or lobby government, our retailers and manufacturers for change, we cannot advocate in our workplaces or talk to our unions,' she told me. 'Wen believes it should not be left up to women to avoid these chemicals. We surely have a right to a healthy environment, all environments, our living and working environment, and our first environment, the womb.' Wen thinks the focus should be on legislators to protect us, and on manufacturers to use a more precautionary approach to ingredients, avoiding their use if there is any indication they could be harmful.

In the meantime, though, what can we as individuals and consumers do to protect both ourselves and the planet, and encourage change by voting with our wallets? The following is a suggestion of a few places to start.

- **Use up what you have** – don't simply chuck away your existing products. Use them up and then make more mindful choices when you replace them.
- **Reduce consumption** – as with food, and as with 'fast fashion', stop participating in a throwaway culture, and try to only buy what you really need.
- **Choose products in reusable or recyclable packaging** – if the brand is being mindful of its impact in this area, it may well also be creating products with fewer nasties.
- **Check ingredients** – just as with UPF, begin to be more aware of what's in your cosmetics and opt for brands with more natural ingredients, if possible. You can use apps to check; I recommend the Yuka app, which gives a quick rating based on the barcode.

- **Support organic brands** – these products only use ingredients grown on organic farms, which in turn are kinder to nature.[41]
- **Look for the EU Ecolabel** – if you're outside the EU, choose cosmetics that are approved and sold in the EU. The EU has the strictest chemical regulations in the world, and so these cosmetics may have fewer harmful chemicals in them.[42]
- **Go reusable or organic with your menstrual products** – toxic chemicals and plastics in pads and tampons are not good for you or the planet, so seek out either disposable, unscented, chlorine-free or organic brands, or switch to reusable options like washable pads or menstrual cups.
- **Leave your vulva in peace!** – don't buy intimate washes, they wreak havoc on your vaginal microbiome and are completely unnecessary. They belong in the bin!
- **Limit fragranced products** – from period pads to candles, we live in a scented world of around 4,000 chemicals, around 1,200 of which have been flagged as potential or known concerns by Women's Voices for the Earth.[43] Again, ask – do I need this?
- **Limit plastics** – reduce your plastic use in as many areas as you can – choose glass or metal storage containers for food as well as cosmetics, and keep plastics out of the microwave and dishwasher, as this can break them down.
- **Lobby for change** – get involved with organizations working to address these issues and do what you can to support them, everything makes a difference, no matter how big or small.

11.

Disrespecting the Mother

How UPF damages the Earth

Nature is female. The Earth is female, too. We think of them both as 'mothers': Mother Nature, Mother Earth. Across cultures, throughout history, and entwined in every myth we find the same image: Gaia, the Greek personification of the Earth and the mother of all life; Pachamama, the Inca's world mother, goddess of fertility and the harvest; Grandmother Spider, the Native American timeless woman, benevolent helper, and weaver of webs; Papa, the Māori Earth Mother who sighs out the mists in sorrow at her separation from Rangi, the sky god. Folklore and stories from around the world depict women, if not as the Earth herself, then as powerful guardians of it: healers, growers, herbalists, protectors, presiders over both fertility and harvest.

As women, this is perhaps an affinity we have forgotten, abandoned by a culture that tells us that God, the source of all creative power, is a man, and that women were not only fashioned from Adam's rib as an afterthought, but then entirely responsible for the loss of the ultimate garden, Eden. We are taught that a male deity created everything, and at the same time taught that having the power to create is 'nothing special', and that our cycles, blood, fertility and milk are, at best, a little outmoded, and at worst, a source of shame. It is this paradox that UPF companies have mirrored and exploited, wearing the archetype of 'mother' like a costume, whilst at the same time telling us that feeding and nurturing and creating are 'old hat' and obsolete. By disguising themselves in their marketing as wholesome mums who bake and as pot-stirring Italian nonnas, the makers of UPF have behaved in ways so exploitative and destructive to the planet they would make even the kindly Grandmother Spider wrap them up in a killer web. As women in a patriarchal world, we may find this mistreatment of Mother Earth relatable, if not at a personal level, then as members of the sex who, globally, are still regularly undervalued, harmed and abused.

Some feminists have chosen to explore these connections between the disrespect of women and the disrespect of the Earth and nature. In a world organized by patriarchy, women and nature are seen not as giver, healer, partner or teacher, but as inferior, weak, easily dominated and exploited. Everything historically associated with men – culture, industry, science, politics – is seen to have greater value than that which we historically associate with women – motherhood, domesticity, plant-lore, nature. That which has lesser value can be viewed as a commodity, mined as a resource, and cast aside once depleted and no longer perceived to be of use. Women's labour and the products of our labour are regarded as being of lesser value, just as the offerings of nature are taken for granted. This approach can be seen throughout much of global history, and extends not just to women and nature but to indigenous peoples and other marginalized groups. Such exploitation is consistently presented as vital to human progress; those who protest it are characterized as ill-informed and regressive. As we consider the issue of our current UPF system, particularly as women, it's interesting to bear some of these ideas in mind, and to think about the parallels between the damage UPF is wreaking on our individual bodies and the damage UPF production is doing to women as a sex class, and to the natural world. We may also consider the role that we as women can play in change, through activism, or in our workplaces, or simply through another denigrated 'feminine' value – caring. The shopping trolley is political: as we each make our individual choices of what to put on our plate, we are also choosing which systems to support, and what kind of future world we desire. Let's take a hard look at the systems and future we are supporting when we choose UPF.

Discarded packaging

I can't be the only person living in a family house (I have three kids) that finds themself aghast at the amount of packaging waste we generate every week. Even though my part of the UK has a fairly extensive recycling programme, it still seems insane to me every time I add another plastic meat tray or sturdily built cardboard Tetra Pak to the pile. The average UK home now throws away around sixty pieces of plastic packaging a week, meaning that as a nation we throw away 90 billion pieces of plastic packaging a year;[1] only in the USA do they produce more plastic waste per person. Only around 9 per cent of plastic waste produced globally is ever recycled; 79 per cent of it ends up in landfills, or in nature.² In 2021, the United Nations Environment Programme estimated that there were 75–199 million tonnes of plastic in our global oceans.³ Plastic waste is causing havoc in the natural world, and so much of it comes from food and drink packaging. A study published in May 2024, in which the labels of millions of discarded plastic items were analysed, found that 11 per cent of the world's plastic waste comes from Coca-Cola, and that 25 per cent of it comes from just five companies: Coca-Cola, Nestlé, PepsiCo, Danone and Altria (formerly Philip Morris).⁴ The scale of this problem is so big that it's easy to forget the other issue with plastic, and these big companies would probably prefer if we did: 99 per cent of plastic is made from chemicals sourced from fossil fuels – the oil industry and the plastic industry are inextricably linked.⁵

Most of us are aware of the environmental impact of the aviation industry, which emitted 426 million tonnes of carbon dioxide equivalent (tCO2e) in 2022. Some even choose not to fly because of this planetary harm. But you might be more surprised to learn that, at 477 million tCO2e, the global emissions of the world's ten biggest food and drink manufacturers in the same year were even higher, according to a new report from Bite Back 2030.⁶ When we choose to eat an apple bar instead of an apple, many of us don't think about the environmental damage of this choice, even if we have perhaps tentatively begun to think of the damage to our own bodies. We have not always lived this way: a trip to a deli counter or a greengrocer or a butcher may remind you of a world, still in living memory, in which we lived without quite so many UPF products and quite so much packaging. My grandad in his shop with his wire cheese slice was, in small ways that add up and count, doing the world a considerable favour. He would not comprehend my overflowing weekly boxes of sorted packaging for the recycling truck nor, since he died in 2000, would he probably ever have encountered another aspect of UPF that is now in every home: palm oil. In 1995, Unilever became the first company to switch to palm oil across its production lines, due to growing health concerns about trans fats. Over the following two decades its use skyrocketed, to the point where it is now in around half of all UPF products, from cookies to pizza to chocolate, as well as so many other household items from shampoo to dog food. This comes at a significant cost.

Discarded trees

Some of you are probably already trying to buy products that don't include palm oil, or that say the palm oil used is 'sustainable'. Many of us were alerted to the issues with palm oil by news of the plight of the orangutan, caused by palm oil production. This was first highlighted by a 2018 advertising campaign by the supermarket Iceland featuring a cartoon baby, 'Rang Tan', which was banned for being too political, and then by footage in David Attenborough's 2019 documentary, *Climate Change: The Facts*, in which an adult orangutan faced off a bulldozer as it razed trees to the ground in Borneo to make way for the production of palm oil. It's estimated that over half of the Indonesian rainforest has been lost, much of it to palm oil. Indonesia is now the world's third biggest greenhouse gas emitter, after China and the USA, and this is solely due to the clearing and draining of carbon-rich peatlands and rainforest destruction.[7] As well as the damage to wildlife and complex ecosystems, indigenous peoples are being displaced – according to Human Rights Watch, palm oil plantations have had a devastating impact on the Ibans in Borneo, and on the Orang Rimba, a semi-nomadic, forest-dependent people in central Sumatra, many of whom are now living in plastic tents, and in abject poverty.[8] The women of these communities have suffered in specific ways: deprived of their ability to pass on intergenerational knowledge and skills, cut off from their income sources of basket- and mat-weaving from forest products, and unable to provide for their children.

Researchers studying the impact of palm oil production on another Indonesian indigenous people, the Dayak Benawen of Borneo, have highlighted another loss: women's role in forest conservation and traditional ecological knowledge, including that of local plant and animal species and their uses, passed down through oral traditions.[9] They have a 'psychological bond with nature and the forest', say the researchers, that they are now struggling to maintain. Those women who take jobs within the palm oil industry are also often exploited – low waged, exposed to hazardous fertilizers and chemicals, and vulnerable to sexual assault.[10] Around the world this pattern is repeated, women in farming and food production are likely to be low waged and denied the chance to own land, with men taking the higher paid jobs and controlling the cash, according to Oxfam.[11]

At the moment, the idea of 'sustainable palm oil' divides people, with some, like the World Wildlife Fund (WWF), saying it is possible and that boycotting may even take away resources from companies trying to do the right thing.[12] The WWF has created a Palm Oil Buyers Score Card which it hopes will put pressure on companies to have true supply chain traceability. Greenpeace, on the other hand, says that the whole idea of 'certified sustainable' palm oil is currently 'a con', describing the Roundtable on Sustainable Palm Oil (RSPO) as being 'as much use as a chocolate teapot'.[13] The Rainforest Alliance is also unconvinced, explaining that many companies who use the RSPO label on their products are still causing widespread rainforest destruction and environmental damage through the clearing and draining of carbon-rich peatlands.[14]

Discarded people

Whether or not you decide to boycott, it could be that giving palm oil our focus is distracting us from a much bigger problem – soy. It's estimated that soya bean production is responsible for nearly five times the deforestation as palm oil.[15] In the UK alone, we import over three million tonnes of soya a year, and both in the UK and globally over three-quarters of all soy produced is fed to animals.[16] If soy, or soy-derived products like soy lecithin, vegetable oil, or hydrolysed vegetable protein are not in your UPF itself, then soy has fed the animal whose product – whether egg-, meat- or milk-based – is in your UPF.

Brazil is the world's largest producer and exporter of soy, and it's estimated that around 20 per cent of the Amazon rainforest has now been lost to the cultivation of this simple bean. Ten million years old and home to 390 billion trees and at least 427 species of mammals, the deforested areas of the Amazon now host mainly one plant, soy, and one animal, the cow; Brazil is also the second largest global producer of beef. Also destroyed in the quest to produce soy and beef is the lesser-known area of the Cerrado, a vast tropical savannah that is home to species such as the jaguar and the endangered maned wolf. As destruction of the Amazon slows in Brazil under the leadership of Lula da Silva, the devastation of the Cerrado seems to be increasing.[17] Such destruction, and the slash-and-burn techniques employed, release large amounts of carbon into the atmosphere, contributing to global warming.

When I was researching probiotic foods like kimchi and sauerkraut (see page 135), I went to visit Paula Neubauer who runs Get Pickled from her home in Somerset, a small business that makes ferments and runs workshops to teach others how to do so. She opened my eyes to the creativity and explosive flavours of her craft, but she also had another story to tell, that of the Guarani-Kaiowá community, an indigenous people from the Mato Grosso do Sul in her native Brazil. She begins by telling me about some serious conflicts of interest in the production of soya:

'We have had Blairo Maggi, a man who is a billionaire and the biggest producer of soy in Brazil, being appointed the Minister of Agriculture. Now we have Carlos Fávaro in that job, who has been President of the Brazilian Soy Producers Association. It's crazy. When you go to Brazil, you can't believe your eyes. The fields of soy stretch as far as the eyes can see, and further, they are so vast you cannot even imagine. If it's not soy, it's corn, which they only plant so that they can claim soy is not a monocrop, and this gets used for corn syrup, which is also in a lot of UPF. They spray on a lot of pesticides, and the cancer rates in children have risen, they are pretty sure it's because of these chemicals in the drinking water.'

A 2023 study unfortunately suggests this is true, showing an additional 123 deaths of children from acute lymphoblastic leukaemia in the Cerrado, where people are exposed to high levels of pesticides in the water supply.[18]

The Guarani-Kaiowá people have been being displaced since cattle farming and soy production began in the mid-twentieth century, in a battle that has often turned bloody – *many* Guarani-Kaiowá have lost their lives in the struggle to face down government evictions and remain on their ancestral lands. Paula's interest in the Guarani is specific – they make a unique fermented drink called chicha – and it's made solely by women:

'The Guarani see men as of the sky and women as of the earth. So women are the sacred guardians of the chicha technique because it is of the earth. Young girls get involved with the women in making chicha from the age of about ten. I think, in many cultures, we have lost touch with what fermentation means as a social and cultural tool, and as a female domain. The Guarani now also stand to lose this traditional knowledge and practice, due to what the UN have called an ethnocide. There's particular hatred towards the women of the Guarani, too. Because there is a very strong born-again Christian element in Brazil now and they see women's wisdom as witchcraft. They burn down their sacred houses. All of this destruction in the name of God, but mostly in the name of soya.'

There are pockets of hope. I spoke to Cynthia Moleta Cominesi, a sustainability consultant who works in Brazil, trying to help strike a balance between the need for economic advancement and the importance of environmental protection. 'I believe we are improving every day in terms of sustainability,' she told me. 'We have no-till farming, precision agriculture, biological control, and the use of drones is advancing significantly. Here in the Cerrado, it is possible to have two harvests, and we also have the crop-livestock-forest integration system.' When she worked with the World Wildlife Fund, Cynthia was involved in a project called 'People Who Produce and Preserve', helping female soy farmers to preserve the forest between the Cerrado and the Amazon Biome and getting the women involved certified by the Round Table on Responsible Soy Association (RTRS). 'Women are the future of responsible soy,' says Cynthia. 'I think women have certain characteristics that make them more likely to support actions related to sustainable development. I believe this is because they are mothers. Personally, I am like that; everything I do, I consider the implications for my children. Therefore, we tend to support initiatives that we know will bring a better future for the next generations.'

Sweet like cola?

Just as food companies have undermined and broken our relationship with real food in the Western world, so too have they turned to developing countries and encouraged their people to associate UPF in plastic packaging with liberation and progress. Doctor and author Chris van Tulleken has documented Brazil's 'Nestlé boat' in his BBC documentary, *What are we feeding our kids?* This floating barge, filled with powdered milk, yoghurt, cookies and sweets, was launched in 2010 and travelled up the Amazon basin, taking these sugary products to remote communities. It's probably unlikely that the packaging from UPF consumed in more remote parts of the world will find its way to a recycling depot, and van Tulleken believes this boat project, known as 'Nestlé Takes You Onboard', also marked the beginning of obesity in this region. 'I have not found any evidence that there were children with diet-related diabetes in these parts of Brazil until enterprises like the Nestlé boat,' he writes in his book, *Ultra-Processed People*. In Brazil, as in the rest of the world, the most frequently purchased beverage is Coca-Cola, and in almost every country of the world, with one or two notable exceptions, it is made with an ingredient called high-fructose corn syrup (HFCS), which comes from another crop that causes widespread environmental damage: maize.

So just in case of confusion, maize and corn are the same thing, and although – as Paula Neubauer explained to me – a fair bit of corn is grown in Brazil, by far the biggest global producer is the USA, followed by China. If you've started looking at UPF packaging, you'll have noticed that maize and modified maize starch are in lots of items, but most of the world's corn is used as animal feed. An aerial view of the Midwest of America, known as the Corn Belt, will paint you a full picture: swathes of maize fields stretch for hundreds of miles alongside barren 'feedlots' where cows are corralled and fattened for market. Cows aren't meant to eat corn, they're ruminants, which means they're meant to eat grass, so the whole process is slightly dystopian. This intensive and unnatural way of farming is causing damage: around 4,300 Americans die a premature death each year due to the air pollution caused by fertilizers and dust from corn production;[19] and water run-off from fertilizers in the Corn Belt is causing algae to bloom in the Gulf of Mexico, choking off oxygen in the water and creating a 'dead zone' the size of New Jersey where nothing will live.[20] Such intensive farming of just one crop is also causing soil erosion in a way that is not without precedent: in the 1930s, millions of tonnes of topsoil blew off the Great Plains and polluted America in an environmental disaster knows as the Dust Bowl. Now, experts say dust levels across the Great Plains are rising year on year, as huge fields with little or no trees make it more difficult for the ground to retain moisture as global temperatures rise.[21] None of these problems is caused by nature; rather they are entirely the fault of human behaviour and corporate greed.

American-made corn syrup does find its way into UK products like biscuits, ice cream and cakes, appearing on labels as 'glucose-fructose syrup'. But much of our sweetness, including in our cola, comes from a different crop – sugar beet.[22] Grown on areas of land in East Anglia and the East Midlands that are equivalent in size to the area devoted to all other vegetable crops put together, sugar beet is then delivered to one of four UK refineries, all owned by British Sugar. Around 1.2 million tonnes of refined sugar are produced annually – two-thirds more than the World Health Organization's (WHO) recommended allowance of sugar per day for a year, for the whole of the UK population combined. This huge demand for sugar is driving soil erosion here, too – when the beet is harvested, the earth clings to the plants, making up around 20 per cent of the 2.9 million tonnes of topsoil the UK loses per year. Nearly 85 per cent of fertile peat soils have been lost in East Anglia since 1850, and the remainder risk being lost over the next thirty years.[23] The UK government has highlighted soil as an overlooked area of environmental policy, stating that intensive agriculture has caused arable soils to lose about 40–60 per cent of their organic carbon. And soil – as much as we may take it for granted as the simple mud under our feet – really matters for our future: we need topsoil to grow around 90 per cent of the world's food. Some experts say if soil erosion continues at current levels, we risk running out of topsoil in less than sixty years.[24] 'We have sixty harvests left,' is their extremely frightening prediction.

Green fingers

As we continue to exploit the ground itself, we forget that our relationship with soil is two-way and that we are what we eat even at a microbial level. We need dirt, and we need the microbes in the dirt. Researchers are now just beginning to explore the relationship between the microbes in soil and the microbes in our guts, and considering the ways in which our depleted soil from aggressive farming practices could be having an impact on our bodies.[25] Good, healthy soil and good healthy humans, it seems, have a symbiotic relationship – our food that is grown in the dirt imparts both nutrition and microbes to our guts, and as we deplete the bacterial diversity of the dirt, so we deplete our own bacterial diversity. It's even thought that we are literally not eating as much dirt as we perhaps should be or used to, as so many of us now live in homes cleaned to a state of sterility and have little or no contact with the soil. If you've ever washed a home-grown carrot or potato, you'll know it's completely different in terms of dirt than the bright shiny versions you get in the shops. And it's likely that a little bit of that dirt, complete with soil microbes, will find its way into your body when you eat, or touch your hands to your face whilst gardening. Researchers have found that in families who have one primary gardener, the gut microbiomes of the whole family contain bacteria from the soil, and that, in gardening season, not just the gardener but the whole family has higher gut microbial diversity, higher fibre intake and greater abundance of fibre-fermenting bacteria compared to families who do not garden.[26]

Some of the world's people actively and deliberately eat soil in a practice known as geophagy, and the most common time for this to happen is during pregnancy and lactation.[27] In sub-Saharan Africa, it's estimated that as many as 84 per cent of pregnant women practise geophagy, most often eating soil with a high clay content, sometimes mixed with herbs.[28] Many say they do this because they crave it, others believe it to have medicinal properties. In the past this behaviour was thought risky and strange, but new understandings of the microbiome suggest it may well be rooted in an older knowledge of the body's needs – although it's still not necessarily something to recommend to pregnant women. In mice, exposure to highly diverse soil dust has been shown to change the gut microbiota with potential mental health benefits.[29] Anyone who has spent time with their hands in the soil will tell you they already knew this. Our soil can save us: we must save it.

Regenerative farming

There's a new approach to the land that has been gathering more attention over the past decade: regenerative farming. Although not formally defined (and therefore ripe for exploitation by UPF companies, which are bound to start waving the word *regenerative* around on their packaging any day now!), it tends to involve a different approach to the soil, for example 'no-till' (mentioned by Cynthia Moleta Cominesi, page 238). This means that the soil is left as undisturbed as possible by keeping digging and ploughing to a minimum, reducing erosion and increasing water retention. Farms are turning to agroecology – sustainable ways of working with nature – methods that are not really 'new' and were often employed by some of the indigenous cultures that ultra-processed agriculture has displaced. For example, symbiotic or companion planting was used by Native Americans, who understood the way that monocropping would deplete soil. Instead, they used the 'three sisters' method, placing squash, maize and beans alongside each other. In her book, *Braiding Sweetgrass*, Robin Wall Kimmerer writes of how indigenous women's knowledge of how the 'three sisters' protect and feed each other, regenerate the soil, and create environments for insect diversity in which the crop-eaters are eaten and kept under natural control, was perceived as ignorance by colonizers. 'To their minds,' she writes, 'a garden meant straight rows of single species, not a three dimensional sprawl of abundance.' When the same colonizers saw plentiful rice harvests and noted how much of the crop was left unreaped, they took this as evidence of laziness, not understanding how strong principles of living in harmony with nature and taking only what you need was key to the plenitude they observed.

In South Somerset, Dawn Quince and her partner, Matt Wade, practise another form of polyculture at their six-acre farm. Dawn told me:

'I became interested in both soil science and agroforestry whilst studying at college. In 2009 I realized a dream and purchased a former tree nursery. Whilst others may have started out by getting rid of the trees, I kept them – there was clearly an ecosystem here and it would have been senseless to destroy it. Agroforestry is the combining of tree crops with livestock or arable, which provides great benefits to the soil, preventing erosion, providing habitats and increasing the microbial diversity, which is good for us humans as well. We focus on making a living growing nutritious salad leaves and slow-grown chicken, whilst building the soil and protecting the wildlife that lives here. We run our chickens under the fruit trees so they get the benefit of the shade and shelter, the fruit trees receive nutrients from the chickens' manure. Any excess manure is composted and used to feed the soil to grow salads. We keep it simple here: no chemical inputs plus tree roots plus organic matter equals healthy soil, which equals healthy food for us and our customers.'

For Dawn, her farm has become a way of life. 'I do it because I can see slow worms and occasional dormice,' she tells me. 'And because, fundamentally, food growing and looking after the planet should co-exist in the same fields. I feel that women are actively engaged in the process of evolution and the bringers of life into this world, so to me it makes sense that we should really be the guardians or spokeswomen for the planet and Mother Nature.'

This kind of attention to nature and soil can be given at an individual level, too. Róisín Nolan was in her late twenties when she started to grow her own vegetables and quickly began to pay particular attention to role of the soil in growing nutrient-dense, high-quality food. 'I'd always had an interest in self-sufficiency,' she told me. 'Then I came across books like *The Intelligent Gardener* by Steve Solomon that made the link between soil and health. Soil is where everything starts.' Róisín is now seven years in to a programme of adding selenium and other nutrients to her veg patch in her native county Limerick, in Ireland, where she grows everything from potatoes to herbs on six plots of 20×20ft with two polytunnels. 'We are completely self-sufficient on things like potatoes, onions, garlic, leeks, scallions, lettuces, cabbages and beets,' she says. 'And we probably buy about half of our tomatoes, cucumbers, chillies and peppers from other local growers and grow the rest. We make our own wild wines, too!'

As far as soil goes, she and her partner, Kieran, spend time and attention making compost based on what the soil needs. 'We need to think more about microbes and how we are influenced by the microbes in the world around us and what we eat,' she explains. 'Even a seed comes with its own microbiome on its coat, which interacts with the soil when planted. This will tell the plant what type of nutrition is available in the soil and this will dictate its growth habits. I have personally found it very rewarding to grow my own food in a way that has such clear health benefits – eating from my garden and locally sourced meats has greatly improved my arthritis.' Róisín is passionate that other people feel empowered to grow their own. 'I started growing veg with peas and parsley in two pots outside my door,' she says. 'How to eat an elephant? One bite at a time. Start small and only grow what you love to eat. It's a learning curve, but one that teaches that we are part of an amazing planet.'

Food companies are beginning to feel pressure to change.

As well as increasing scrutiny as the world wakes up to these issues, there is also no profit to be made from soil in which nothing will grow. Ignoring and disrespecting nature is a bit of a spectacular self-own for those whose livelihoods depend on her bounty. In Brazil, for example, researchers have used the term 'agro-suicide' to describe the way that deforestation has affected rainfall, causing soy yields to decrease.[30] If you ask the big food companies what they are doing about all this, they have plenty of answers, but it's hard to discern how much is lip-service and green-washing, and how much is genuinely going to enact change. Many UPF companies use similar phraseology, 'We are striving to reduce our footprint', 'We care about our impact', and so on.[31] Coca-Cola, for example, says it is working to end plastic pollution, pledging to make 100 per cent of its packaging recyclable globally by 2025, and to use at least 50 per cent recycled material in packaging by 2030. But 'making packaging recyclable' does not mean it will be recycled, particularly not in parts of the world where such services are inaccessible. I contacted Coca-Cola to ask for more information about how they hoped to end plastic pollution, but they did not respond. There are many organizations working to persuade food companies to take action, and some of them are in Resources section on page 309 if you want to support them. But, while we wait for them to change, I truly believe we can reduce our own personal impact on the planet and, more than that, actually make a positive difference – by changing what we put on our plates.

Regenerative eating

As shoppers, cooks and consumers, we *can* make a difference. If you are reading this book, you are already on a path to change, and this can involve not just a focus on your own body or the health of yourself and your loved ones, but a realization of the interconnectedness of humans, nature and the Earth, and that physical health, mental health, gut health, soil health, animal health, and the health of the planet itself all impact each other and matter to each other. This sense of interconnectedness has been lost in the aisles of plastic-wrapped products. Shifting your focus and becoming more mindful of the impact on the planet of your food choices is bound to transform the way that you shop and eat – and you will definitely do the best you can in whatever ways are possible and accessible to you, and this *will* make a difference. Small changes add up.

We have come to rely on UPF and to see it as integral to our lives, but slowly, at a pace we can manage, we need to turn this thinking around. We have to accept that our consumption of UPF is driving industrialized farming and planetary damage that could be catastrophic for future generations. As we look at labels, we can start to notice the ubiquitous soya, sugars and palm oil and ask ourselves if we can make swaps. Every small change will make a difference. If everyone who reads this book simply swapped out cola and fizzy drinks and replaced them with water, this alone would help. We can then progress up the Pyramid of Change (see page 251) and begin to ask, 'do I really need this food?', making a few more swaps. Gradually, we may progress to the 80/20 approach, where we have some UPF in our diet but are cooking a lot more wholefoods from scratch.

Beyond this, we may begin to think about the meat we buy, not just in terms of animal welfare (which is important), but also in terms of planet welfare. Grass-fed and organic meat is more expensive – but can we eat meat less often and focus on planet welfare when we do? For some, the UPF journey will end with a situation of zero tolerance, or even what I have named on the pyramid 'Utopia', an unlikely but possible situation in which we know the story of every food item in our fridge and cupboards. This may not be possible for most of us, but even the 'small swaps' approach will make a difference. We can all do our best.

In doing so, we will help with the planet regeneration that is currently needed. I feel like I've always been given the impression that this intensive agriculture is necessary to provide enough food for everyone on the planet, but this simply isn't the case. At the moment, roughly one-third of food produced for human consumption is lost or wasted globally – and this amounts to about 1.3 billion tonnes per year.[32] And around one-third of global arable land is used to produce feed for livestock, mainly intensively farmed animals, rather than for humans directly.[33] I asked Rob Percival, Head of Food Policy for the Soil Association, if a new way is possible. 'Yes,' he answered definitively. 'Put very simply, if we wasted less food, and used land to feed humans directly instead of animals in factory farms, we would have plenty to go around.' He pointed me to a European study.[34] 'This shows that organic or nature-friendly farming – without chemical and synthetic inputs, and with high levels of animal welfare – could feed a growing population a healthy diet, while also making space for nature recovery and carbon capture – with the feasibility of the scenario contingent on a little less waste and diets including roughly 50 per cent less meat.'

So there is hope and possibility of change, but the current picture is bleak. As a woman, the exploitation of our planet is unfortunately relatable. I know what it's like to feel unheard or disrespected; at times in my life this has been because I was perceived as beautiful and fertile; at other times because I was perceived as barren or depleted; but in both cases it was entirely because I am female. In my work campaigning for better birth experiences I have heard a thousand stories of women being treated as if they had no feelings, physical or emotional, as they cross the threshold to motherhood. As a therapist in my twenties and thirties, I held space for many women and children who were victims of male violence or other misogynistic acts. I have lost count of the number of female friends who have felt, from time to time, or most of the time, mistreated, disrespected and used. And now in my forties, this only seems to intensify as myself and those same friends hit menopause and feel invisible and as though the gifts we have given have been taken for granted. When I think about the way we are damaging our planet, I can't help but see parallels, and long for a new world order in which regeneration, rather than exploitation, is held to be essential to progress; in which both female people and the Earth herself are cherished and respected as our vital life source. Whether or not you see these parallels, I'm pretty sure that as you come to the end of this book, you'll agree that our current way of going about things cannot be sustained.

For our bodies, for women, for the planet, and for the future, there has to be a better way.

Pyramid of Change

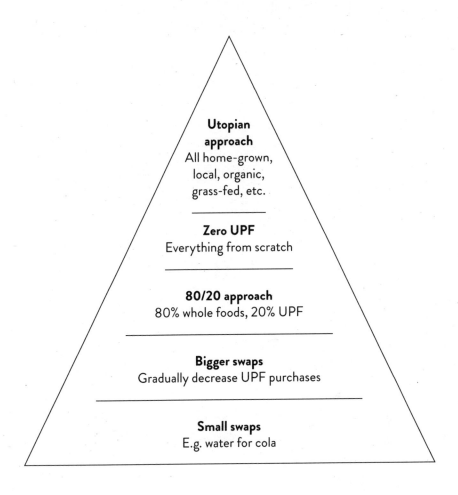

12.

Seeds of change

How to quit or reduce UPF

As I've researched and written this book, I've gone on my own journey with UPF, and begun to learn more about the ways in which this food has become embedded in my kitchen cupboards, my family meals, my snack choices, and my shopping trolley. I've also had many, many conversations with both real-life friends and women who have got in touch online in which the key question has been, 'what is UPF?', and then, 'how do I stop eating it?' And in between those two questions, there is often a journey, similar to the one I've taken myself, in which people move thorough various stages of shock, denial and bargaining, eventually moving towards acceptance. The fact is, most of us don't like to think we are eating much UPF at all. We all like to think we eat healthily, and it can come as a surprise to realize that UPF is not just McDonald's, but something that has crept stealthily into all of our cupboards, fridges and freezers. There are some UPF foods that really shocked me – that tin of coconut milk that I happily pour into a homemade curry, not realizing it's full of gums and emulsifiers, those posh crisps I keep in the cupboard for when a friend drops round for a drink, that 'plant-based' milk I give my son with allergies, those tubs of expensive ice cream.

So this section of the book is a compendium of thoughts, ideas and practical suggestions, intended to help anyone who has reached that place of realization and acceptance and is now thinking about reducing the amount of UPF in their own or their family's diet, or even trying to cut it out completely. I've included as much 'entry-level' advice as I can, because I know that many of us are feeling completely deskilled in the kitchen and need to go back to basics. I've also included a few really simple recipes that I hope will encourage you to see just how quick and easy it can be to make your own food. Over time, we need policy-makers and people with power to help the world make big changes in our approach to the food in our shops, but in the meantime, people need to know what to make for dinner tonight, and how. I guess it's important to say, too, that just because this chapter contains practical advice about shopping and cooking, I am not for a second implying that this is 'women's work'. Changing away from UPF is everyone's business and everyone's job. I hope the excitement of a busy kitchen, filled with fantastic new smells, tastes and textures, becomes contagious in your household – may it be a place where everyone is happy and everyone pulls their weight.

One more thing: this chapter is entirely focused on UPF, and therefore it doesn't contain any other kind of dietary advice. If you want to lose weight, or go vegan, or build muscle, or make sure your kids are getting the right nutrients, you need a different book. I really think it's important, when we tackle the UPF problem, to stick to the brief. There are conversations to be had about organic food, the dairy industry, meat, fats, sugar…it can get complex. Our goal here is just to focus on UPF, because I think it's the single biggest positive change you can make for your health. Once you make the change away from UPF, you might get curious about other dietary questions, and there are other resources that will help you out with this. Today, let's just think about removing as much UPF from your diet as possible and replacing it with wholefoods, packed with nutrients. The rest will fall into place as sure as eggs are eggs.

Is it UPF or not?

If you pick up a jar of sauce or a box of biscuits, you are going to have to start asking this question before you put it in your trolley. I highly recommend you download an app called Open Food Facts, which allows you to scan the barcode and will give you a rating for the most common products. However, it's best to use your own brain as well. Flip over the box or packet and look at the ingredients. Ask yourself:

- **What is in this food?**
- **Do I recognize all the ingredients as food?**

If you are trying to completely cut out UPF and it contains ingredients that don't sound like food, for example emulsifiers, gums, E numbers, names that sound like they belong in a science lab, etc., then put it back on the shelf.

If you are going for a more moderate approach, then you could also ask:

- **Is this food? Or is it a factory-made 'formulation'?**

Remember – to be counted as Group 4 and therefore UPF under the Nova classification (see page 20), the food needs to be a 'formulation, made mostly or entirely from substances derived from foods and additives, with little if any intact Group 1 food'. For example, a tin of kidney beans that contains a 'firming agent' is not Nova 4, and not UPF. The beans are still intact and recognizable as a Group 1 food, but have been processed by being canned with an additive, and therefore fall into Group 3, a 'processed food'. If they're canned without any additives, they are arguably Group 1, 'minimally processed'. A packet of biscuits, on the other hand, with a list of ingredients as long as your arm that goes way beyond the required ingredients for a biscuit (sugar, butter, flour and maybe egg), is a 'formulation', made with shelf-life and uniformity and profit in mind, not nutrition. It might look like a biscuit, but it's actually faking it.

If you decide that you don't want to eat any foods that contain firming agents or additives of any kind, this is a valid choice, but it's perhaps unhelpful to mix this in with the idea of cutting out UPF, especially for people on a budget or who don't have the time to shop around for completely organic, additive-free products. The problem with true UPF is that it's low in fibre, low in nutrients, hyperpalatable, calorie dense, moreish and addictive. None of this is true of a tinned kidney bean. My own approach is to think about the benefits of a home-cooked meal and, even if there are one or two additives in my raw ingredients, not to let concern about ultra-processing tip over into anxiety about food, for me or my family. A big bowl of chilli made with beans that contain a firming agent is far better than a microwave meal or a takeaway. Overall, I think it's okay 'not to sweat the small stuff', but your approach might be different. I guess another way of thinking about it could be:

- Do I really need this food?

'Need' is a personal thing. It means you will have to balance the benefit of that particular food item to you, the practicality of alternatives, the cost, how much time you have, and the level of 'nasties' on the label, and make a considered decision. For example, if you are absolutely exhausted, on your way home from work with a toddler you just picked up from nursery who is screaming and refusing to get in the trolley, then you might feel the benefits of a quick frozen pizza outweigh any negatives. Even then (if the toddler will allow), it's worth having a quick look through the different frozen pizzas on offer, because some brands are worse than others. You could try the Open Food Facts app in this situation – if you've got enough hands free. I would definitely advise a nuanced approach, and one that doesn't make life impossible or suck all the joy out of cooking and eating. Instead, allow these new UPF ideas to set you on a culinary journey, with a love of good food at its heart.

Changing what goes in the trolley

The key to moving away from UPF is to make a conscious effort to buy as many single-ingredient foods as you can and feed yourself and your family from them. Some examples of single-ingredient foods you might want to put regularly in your trolley are:

- fruit (fresh, frozen or tinned);
- vegetables (fresh, frozen or tinned);
- onions;
- tinned tomatoes and passata (the latter is just puréed, sieved canned tomatoes);
- oil (olive, if possible);
- herbs and spices (see page 287);
- meat (fresh or frozen);
- fish and seafood (tinned, fresh or frozen);
- eggs;
- beans, pulses and lentils (tinned or dried);
- potatoes;
- pasta;
- rice;
- cheese;
- natural yoghurt;
- oats (porridge);
- nuts;
- seeds;
- flour;
- butter;
- sugar.

Some examples of simple meals you can make from the above list:

- macaroni or cauliflower cheese;
- fish, rice and salad or vegetables;
- pasta with a homemade sauce;
- tray-roasted chicken thighs with roasted vegetables;
- homemade pizza;
- jacket potatoes topped with tuna / cheese / beans with veg or salad;
- Bolognese sauce;
- stew / casserole;
- soup.

Basic kitchen equipment

This is something you can build on as you get more into cooking, but as a starter-kit I would say you need something like:

- one frying pan;
- one or two saucepans;
- one roasting tin;
- one or two baking trays, approx. 33×22cm;
- one wooden spoon;
- one spatula
- one small chopping knife and one big one
- set of chopping boards;
- colander or sieve;
- oven gloves.

The size of the pans depends on how many people you are feeding, but even if you are cooking for one, a 4-litre or 5-litre saucepan will be useful for batch-cooking something like Bolognese or soup and freezing portions. It will also be useful for making stock. If your budget is tight, you can usually get many of the above items from charity shops.

I also find a stick blender to be an absolutely brilliant gadget. The one I have comes with different attachments – a whisk, two different-sized pots (the little one is good for making breadcrumbs, chopping garlic, etc., and the big one is good for things like hummus, smoothies and milkshakes), and then the 'stick' part that you can use to blend soup directly in the saucepan – so easy. The better quality brands are fairly expensive but the last one I bought lasted at least fifteen years, so it was value for money.

Shop local

You may not have time to make jam, pickle, chutney or kimchi yourself, but try to find out if there is someone in your local area who is doing this. That roadside stall you pass on your way back from the train station could give you the most flavoursome marmalade of your life, and at the same time help you to cut down on the supermarket versions of these kitchen staples, most of which are UPF. You'll also be supporting an individual human, local to you, rather than Big Food. It's a win all round.

It's also worth investigating other local options, for example small independent shops and local bakeries. Not all bakeries are high-priced and 'artisan'. In my area we have a fantastic bakery called Bakery Roy-Al, where Roy and Al make all sorts of proper loaves of bread without the great long list of additives you'll find in the supermarket brands. They don't make much sourdough, but the bread they do make contains no nasties, and that's good enough for me.

Local butchers will also give you advice on how to cook the various cuts of meat they offer, and local greengrocers may have seasonal fruit and vegetables of better quality than the supermarket. But only do what your time and budget will allow – it's reducing UPF that's the key, and if that means shopping carefully in your budget supermarket, that's fine.

A typical day – without UPF

Let's travel slowly thorough a standard eating day and look at the main meals and snacks, including what you might be eating that is UPF, perhaps without realizing, and then we'll look at how to make changes.

Breakfast

This is an absolutely great place to start your reduction in UPF consumption. At least three-quarters of people in the UK and the USA start their day with boxed cereals, and they are almost all UPF. The worst offenders are the ones that are obviously sugary or chocolatey, designed to look like cookies or even given names like 'Krave' – the clue that they are moreish and addictive is literally on the box! Many are eye-wateringly high in sugar and salt, in particular if you are inclined to eat more than just a very small bowl of them. Any health claims on the packaging can usually be ignored – they may be 'fortified with iron' or similar, but nutrition is more complex than ingesting single, isolated nutrients. Your body wants wholefoods, that often have combinations of nutrients that work together to be absorbed and to do you good. There are a few boxed cereals that, although they are highly processed, don't 'technically' count as UPF, so you can always keep a box of them in the cupboard for back-up.

If it helps break the spell, you might like to know that Kellogg, the man largely responsible for us all starting our days with Corn Flakes, was a bit of an oddball. He somehow managed to merge religion with the matter of breakfast, and was particularly concerned about masturbation, to the point that he employed some horrifyingly medieval methods on the young boys and girls attending his sanatorium to rid them of this practice. He also felt that meat-eating was a cause of masturbation, and it was this that inspired him to come up with the first breakfast cereal, a type of ground-up biscuit he called *granula*. Somehow the marketing of this concept evolved and now we find ourselves at a point where breakfast and a bowl of cereal are inextricably associated, even if cereal and masturbation are not.

You may not fancy the idea of meat for breakfast, but even so, try to rethink this meal completely and move away from the cultural norm of UPF cereal followed by UPF toast. Many other cultures do not eat this stuff! In other parts of the world, it's common to find a combination of eggs, plants, bread, rice, meat and fish, cooked and served in a variety of ways. Often people reheat and re-season the meal from the night before – for example, in Indonesia, a popular breakfast dish is nasi goreng. This is made with last night's leftover rice, fried with onion, garlic, chilli and spices, flavoured with a special sauce called kecap manis (a sweet soy sauce), and topped with a fried egg and a side order of cucumber. In Vietnam they start the day with pho, a spicy soup made with noodles and meat in a rich bone broth. In North Africa you may find shakshuka, a dish of eggs poached in a spicy tomato sauce that, almost certainly owing to its sheer deliciousness, has travelled through Europe and morphed into dishes like huevos a la flamenca, made in Spain with eggs and a spicy chorizo sauce. In Mexico you might find huevos rancheros, and get your eggs and tomato with a side order of refried beans, avocado and fresh coriander. Eggs are a popular breakfast item throughout the world, and for good reason – they are cheap, readily available, and highly nutritious. Across Europe, bread and pastries are also a typical way to start the day, although often in the UK and USA these have evolved from a simple, wholesome product into a textbook example of UPF. If you are buying any kind of breakfast item from the shops, even a simple croissant, you will need to check the ingredients.

Here are some non-UPF breakfasts you could try.

- smashed avocado on toast (see page 276 on bread) with a poached egg on top. Season with chilli flakes, salt and pepper.
- porridge topped with fruit (frozen, tinned or fresh).
- homemade muesli – make your own mix of oats, nuts, seeds, dried fruit.

- Greek yoghurt or kefir (fermented yoghurt), topped with fruit, nuts, seeds.
- halloumi, mushrooms, tomatoes, eggs and toast.
- omelette with any filling (ham, cheese, broccoli, mushroom – so many choices!).
- a simple version of shakshuka – tin of tomatoes in the frying pan over a medium heat, a teaspoon of smoked paprika, make a well in the sauce and drop in an egg until cooked.
- pancakes, sweet or savoury.

In our house the kids have a pancake for breakfast almost every school day. They are so quick and easy to make and if you look online, you'll find infinite variations, including vegan options, American pancakes (the fat, round, fluffy variety), and another of our favourites, banana pancakes.

EASY PANCAKES

100g self-raising flour
300ml milk
2 eggs
a knob of butter or oil for frying

Whisk the ingredients together in a mixing bowl and fry one by one in a large frying pan, for a minute or two per side, until golden. Add your toppings of choice, from cheese to lemon, honey to fruit. This recipe will make eight to twelve pancakes, depending on the size of your pan. To make less, halve the recipe.

Snacking

There's an argument to say that snacking is a concept we've all been sold by the UPF companies and that if we were eating more nutritious meals, they would sustain us for longer, keep our blood sugar on a more even keel, and we wouldn't need extra food in between them. On the other hand, it's possible that eating little and often is a good way to go, and it's certainly better than letting yourself get really hungry and then making 'bad' food choices. Whichever way you choose to eat, it's undeniable that the 'snack aisle' of the supermarket is jam-packed with UPF: crisps, chocolate, snack bars, biscuits and cakes. So if you do want to nibble on something in between meals, it's best to avoid all this stuff and instead try:

- nuts (plain or lightly salted rather than honey roasted, dry roasted or flavoured);
- fruit or veg, e.g. carrot sticks, celery sticks, slices of bell pepper, perhaps with nut butter or homemade hummus – or just an old-fashioned apple or banana!;
- dark chocolate.

There are also lots of really simple snacks that you can make yourself from online recipes. For example:

- granola bars, flapjacks, nut and seed bars;
- nut balls or date balls;
- nuts or fruit, like strawberries, in dark chocolate;
- dates, e.g. stuffed with peanut butter and dipped in dark chocolate;

- biscuits and cookies (really quick and easy to make);
- homemade hummus or mashed avocado with non-UPF crispbread or crackers (you can also make your own crackers, see below;
- if you have to have that bag of crisps, the only ones that are not UPF are ready salted (potato, sunflower oil (see page 290), salt), or you can make your own crisps – lots of recipes online.

EASY HUMMUS

Some shop-bought hummus contains extras or is made with cheaper oils, so for the real thing, it's easy and fun to make your own. There are a gazillion variations, too, on this classic recipe, from beetroot, to pea, to spicy – you can find them all online. Great with breadsticks, carrot sticks, apple slices or tortilla chips.

1 × 400g tin of chickpeas, drained and rinsed
1 garlic clove, crushed
Juice of 1 lemon
2 tablespoons tahini
2 tablespoons olive oil
½ teaspoon ground cumin
A grind of salt and pepper

Put the ingredients in your blender and whizz them up until smooth. If it's a bit thick and sticky, add a little splash of water and pulse again. Repeat this until you reach your desired texture.

EASY CRACKERS

I wanted a cracker recipe that didn't require any faff or special ingredients. I always have these ingredients in the house because I put them in my breakfast most days, and it turns out they made a fantastic, easy cracker.

½ cup milled flaxseed (also called linseed)
½ cup mixed seeds
½ cup oats
Good grind of salt

Pre-heat the oven to 150°C/130°C fan/gas 2 and line a baking tray with baking paper. Combine the seeds, oats and salt in a bowl and add water a few splashes at a time until mixed to a gloopy paste, then spread thinly on a baking tray approx. 35cm. Bake for 45–60 minutes, until golden brown and crispy. Allow to cool and then snap into rough shapes and serve with hummus or cheese. Makes around sixteen to twenty uneven crackers.

Lunch

Lunch is a great opportunity to eat another lovely helping of wholefoods and plants. If you're working from home, like me, you might find this easier because you've got access to your full fridge and kitchen set-up. If you're out of the house, you might have to give it a bit more thought.

Work / college lunches

If you eat lunch at work or college, then you might wish to avoid canteen or café lunches, depending on what they serve, and you definitely want to avoid fast-food restaurants and supermarket or chain-store sandwiches. Instead, you could try homemade salads: think about adding drained and rinsed tinned chickpeas, beans or lentils; tinned mackerel or tuna; hard-boiled eggs; leftover chicken; grated cheese; cottage cheese; feta cheese; walnuts; mixed seeds; cold pasta or rice – along with whatever chopped salads you have: bagged salad leaves; lettuce; cucumber; tomato; avocado; fresh herbs, e.g. mint, parsley, coriander; chopped apple; grated carrot; sliced orange; celery; bell peppers, etc. You can also throw in other leftovers, for example roast potatoes or vegetables, whatever takes your fancy. If you have a microwave at work, you could reheat leftovers there or try advancing into the territory of soups.

Making soup

Quite a lot of tinned soup is UPF, and although the fresh ones in the chilled section can be a bit better, they are expensive. Soup is one of those foods that, once you've realized how cheap and easy it is to make, you will never look back. IT IS JUST THINGS YOU LIKE TO EAT, PUT IN WATER AND BLENDED!

To make soup, always start by peeling, chopping and frying an onion – in olive oil, if possible, but any other oil will do. Adding a little salt at this point will help your onions not to burn, because it draws out the water. Then you just add your other ingredients, whatever they may be, and water or stock.

You will find lots of recipes online, but it's really easy – the idea is just to cook everything until it's easy to blend. Cook for 20–30 minutes until it's all softened, allow to cool slightly and then blend it in the saucepan with your stick blender. If you make extra, you can freeze portions for another day (see batch-cooking, page 299). There are so many recipes for soup online – one of our family favourites is leek and potato, which will even make a mid-week supper if you serve it with grated cheese and crispy bacon bits to go on top, or some leftover chicken, or some hard-boiled eggs, and some nice crusty bread with lashings of real butter. In the winter, spicy soups are lovely, for example with ginger or chilli, and if you add beans, they are a great way to pack in those wonderful legumes. For example, this one is so simple:

SPICY BEAN SOUP

1 tablespoon oil for frying
1 onion, chopped
1 clove of garlic, chopped (if you have it, or use powdered)
1 × 400g tin tomatoes
1 × 400g tin kidney beans, drained and rinsed
Salt, pepper, chilli powder

Fry the onion and garlic in the oil over a medium heat with a sprinkle of salt until soft, then add the tinned tomatoes, the kidney beans, and a little more salt and pepper, and chilli powder. How much? Depends on how hot you like it! So, anything from a quarter to a whole teaspoon. Cook on a medium heat for 5–10 minutes, blend with a stick blender until it's a little bit textured and not completely smooth, serve with chilli flakes, grated cheese or a dollop of natural yoghurt, and crusty bread. Obviously, if you are cooking for more people, you will need more tins of tomatoes and beans, and you will need to up your seasoning accordingly (but you probably won't need more onion unless you get up to about triple the number of tins. (In fact, if you don't have an onion at all, you can still make it, and it will still be nice.)

Or try this other simple one:

BROCCOLI AND WHITE BEAN SOUP

1 tablespoon oil for frying
1 onion, chopped
1 garlic clove, chopped
1 head of broccoli, florets and stalk roughly chopped
800ml chicken or vegetable stock (see page 271)
1 × 400g butter or cannellini beans, drained and rinsed
Salt and pepper

Fry the onion in the oil in a big saucepan over a medium heat. Bung in the garlic, broccoli (you can include the stalk, too, just take the dry end off and peel the outer skin, if you like, as this can be a bit stringy, or leave it on if this doesn't bother you as it's good fibre!). Add the stock and simmer for about 20 minutes over a medium heat, until the broccoli is soft, then add the beans, season, and whizz with a stick blender.

The problem of stock cubes

Stock cubes are one of those ubiquitous kitchen cupboard ingredients that most of us bung into dishes without really asking what's in them. Unfortunately, many of them contain palm oil, maltodextrin (an ultra-processed starchy powder that has been shown to affect gut bacteria and the intestinal barrier[1]), MSG, and other UPF ingredients. So, when it comes to stock cubes, here are your choices.

- Choose one that has the least UPF and decide not to sweat the small stuff (see page 300). For example, some brands' only UPF ingredient is palm oil. Considering you are going to add this to a nutritious bowl of homemade soup or stew, brimming with fibre and micronutrients, you may feel like this is 'good enough'.
- Seek out ready-made, non-UPF stock options. They do exist. Some shops sell them in their frozen or refrigerated section, or in jars. Check the ingredients.
- Use an alternative to stock, for example miso paste (which also comes in UPF versions by the way, so read the label!).
- Don't use any stock. Just rely on the flavours from whatever you are cooking and add a little more seasoning.
- Make your own stock. There are recipes online, of course, but again, it's pretty basic.

HOMEMADE STOCK

If you roast a chicken, or even cook a few drumsticks or thighs, get a big pot, fill it with water, and put the bones or carcass in with one or more of the following: a few peppercorns, a couple of bay leaves, a carrot, an onion, a few cloves of garlic, a stick of celery or two, a few sprigs of fresh herbs like parsley, thyme and rosemary. Then you need to simmer it, preferably with a lid on, on a low heat for about three or four hours. Skim off any scum from the surface occasionally and top up with water if needed. You can do the same with a beef bone, and you can also make vegetable stock by leaving out the meat and upping the veg, and reducing the cooking time to about one hour. Some people keep items like the trimmings from vegetables in a bowl in the fridge and then use them for stock rather than binning them.

Once you've cooked it for the required time, strain it and that's your stock. You can then freeze it, writing on the bag the volume so that you can then just add it to your recipe. You can buy purpose-made freezer bags or just save any bread bags and reuse them for freezing. If freezer space is an issue, once you've strained it you can boil it down to about one-quarter of the original quantity before freezing, and then re-add the water when you come to use it.

Kids' packed lunches

This is a tricky one, because the 'norm' is a big box of UPF and kids don't tend to take kindly to a feta cheese, beetroot and bulgur wheat salad. Hot school dinners are another whole minefield and can often, unfortunately, be UPF or poor quality as well. But here are a few ideas:

- sandwiches (see page 276 on bread);
- pasta salads (e.g. cold pasta bows, tuna, sweetcorn, drizzle of olive oil, seasoning);
- breadsticks or non-UPF crackers/crispbreads, homemade hummus;
- frittata (cold sliced boiled potatoes and whisked egg, baked in an ovenproof dish for 20–30 minutes);
- hard-boiled egg for them to peel themselves;
- rice pot with cold chicken and peas;
- cubes of cheese, carrot sticks and apple slices;
- piece of fruit (avoid dried fruit as this can stick to teeth and cause decay);
- pots of cherry tomatoes or baby cucumbers;
- ready salted crisps (see page 30);
- a small container with two or three tablespoons of natural yoghurt, you can also add frozen blueberries, raspberries, or chopped frozen strawberries, these will keep the yoghurt cool and will have defrosted by lunch. Personally, I also wouldn't feel guilty about adding a sprinkle of sugar, or a dollop of honey or maple syrup, if this makes your child more convinced about it all. For context, there are 4g of sugar in a 'Frubes' (they're those plastic tubes of fruit yoghurt) and over 5g in a Munch Bunch Squashums (they're the ones shaped like strawberries). That's a good teaspoonful – and about 8 per cent of their overall makeup;
- plain homemade cupcake (see recipe coming up).

Making cakes

I don't think I had ever made a cake until I was about thirty years old and I was shocked by how easy it was. Shop-bought cakes are absolutely full of UPF – palm oil and other types of oil, preservatives, syrups, emulsifiers and gums – which is why you can stick them in the cupboard and they'll still be fine to eat in a week or two, probably even a month. Homemade cakes don't last anywhere near that long, but that shouldn't be a problem because they'll probably get eaten within about twenty-four hours. The absolute simplest and easiest cakes to make are cupcakes, and they are great for lunchboxes and kids' parties. Once you've got the knack, you can progress to 'loaf cakes', also super easy, and before you know it you'll be making a Victoria sponge for your local bake off.

SIMPLE CUPCAKES

You'll need a cupcake tray and some paper cupcake cases. This makes twelve cupcakes.

120g self-raising flour
120g butter, at room temperature
120g caster sugar
2 eggs
1 teaspoon vanilla extract
1 tablespoon milk, if needed

Pre-heat the oven to 180°C/160°C fan/gas 4. Put your cupcake cases into the cupcake tray. You can use a mixer if you like and, if you do, you just bung all the ingredients into the mixer and whizz together. I like to do it the old-fashioned way, maybe it's a bit like Betty Crocker's 'adding an egg' (see page 65), I just feel a bit more involved! So if you're not using a mixer, you have to 'cream' the butter and sugar together with a wooden spoon in a large mixing bowl. 'Creaming' is really important because after you've added the flour, you want to be much more gentle with the cake batter – beat the flour too much, and you end up with a rubbery cake. You need the butter at room temperature (I sometimes give it a quick blast in the microwave to soften), then you beat the sugar into the butter until it changes colour from yellow to a creamy white (hence 'creaming'). Once you have lots of air in this butter and sugar mixture, add the eggs and beat them in, add the vanilla, then add the flour and mix gently. If the mixture seems too dry, add a spoon or two of milk. Dollop a bit of the mix in each cupcake case, trying to get it as even as possible, and bake for 15–20 minutes. To tell if any cake is cooked, poke a sharp knife into the centre. If it comes out clean, it's done. Leave to cool (you can put them on a wire rack if you have one), and then that's that! You can ice them once cool if you like, but my family prefers them plain, and obviously, for a lunch box, buttercream icing would be a bit tricky!

Biscuits / cookies

Biscuits are even easier to make yourself than cakes. If someone phones you up and says, 'I'm coming round for a cuppa, I'll be there in twenty minutes,' you can literally have biscuits ready by the time they've arrived and taken off their coat. They are just butter, sugar and flour, and sometimes egg. And once you compare this to the ingredients of standard shop biscuits and cookies – almost all of them contain things like palm oil and emulsifiers – it's definitely worth cutting them out or cutting down on them. Yes, it's harder to have homemade biscuits always to hand, but arguably, we are not built to have biscuits always to hand. Better to have them as an occasional treat.

BASIC COOKIES

110g butter
55g caster sugar
135g plain flour

Pre-heat the oven to 180°C/160°C fan/gas 4 and line a baking tray with baking paper. Cream the butter and sugar until white and fluffy, just like you do in the cupcake recipe. Add the flour, and be gentle with it. Roll the mixture into about twelve balls, roughly the same size, and splodge them onto the baking paper (try to use an eco-friendly baking paper if you can). Bake in the oven for 10–15 minutes. You can also do them in a mixer, if you prefer, mixing the butter and sugar first, then adding the flour. To this basic mix you can add chocolate chips, vanilla, nuts, cinnamon, whatever takes your fancy. This makes twelve cookies.

Okay, let's talk about bread

I actually think bread is the biggest nightmare of all if you are trying to cut out UPF. It's such a big part of most of our lives that it's very hard to stop eating it completely, especially if we have a busy family life. As it's present in at least one, sometimes two or even three meals of our days, it doesn't fall into the 'don't sweat the small stuff' category (see page 300). It's also, in many cases, absolutely packed with UPF ingredients – just take five minutes next time you're in the supermarket to look at the long lists of emulsifiers, preservatives, oils and other unidentifiable stuff on the packaging of the leading brands. Extraordinary, really, when you think that bread is just flour, water, yeast and salt. But when you make it like that, it doesn't last anywhere near as long, it's more unpredictable in appearance and texture, and…well…it's actually a completely different product, isn't it?! So we have all come to accept the uniform, spongy-textured, soft and moreish industrially produced sliced loaves – labelled as 'bread' – as bread (for more on the loose definition of bread, see page 28).

But if you want to reduce or quit UPF, you absolutely have to address the bread question, so here are a few suggestions of how you might tackle it, in order of most taxing to least.

- **Make your own sourdough:** this is the top-tier approach, with the steepest learning curve. Sourdough is bread made with a live 'sourdough starter' – a fermenting mix of flour and water. This gives it a different nutritional quality to bread made with added yeast. There are lots of instructional videos online if you want to go down this

route. Although the actual 'hands on' time of making sourdough isn't huge, it does require some planning as the work of making the loaf is stretched out over two days.
- **Make your own (non-sourdough) bread:** this is a bit simpler, just making bread using the sachets of fast-action dried yeast or even without, such as soda bread. You can do it by hand (therapeutic and satisfying, but takes time) or use a bread-making machine.
- **Buying 'proper' sourdough:** if you have a local artisan baker, chances are they will be making sourdough daily. This is an option if you have the budget for it, as it is usually fairly costly per loaf and it doesn't last very long, on account of the lack of all the UPF preservatives! If you don't think you'll use it all in time, you can always slice it and freeze it, taking out a slice when needed.
- **Buying 'proper' bread:** some bakeries, like my local Bakery Roy-Al, are not into all the fancy artisan stuff and you're likely to get some seriously good bread from them. It may not be made with live cultures and kneaded on the thigh of a bearded hipster, but it still tastes bloody good and contains fewer additives than the supermarket stuff.
- **Sourfaux:** there's a bit of snobbery about supermarket sourdough – some call it 'sourfaux' because it's mass-produced and some of it isn't even made with live yeast, as sourdough technically should be. But at the end of the day, a lot of the supermarket sourdoughs are actually pretty good on the UPF front, and more affordable than loaves from a bakery.

- **Supermarket bakery bread:** as with the 'sourfaux', there are some decent loaves in supermarket bakeries that don't contain any nasties, but you do need to check the ingredients as some contain palm oil, dextrose and other things that don't belong in bread.
- **Mass-produced sourdough:** there's an increasing market for sliced bread, rolls, etc., that are UPF-free. Have a look and see if your local supermarket stocks any of these emerging brands. (The big one in the UK is called Jason's.)

I think, whatever you do, there are going to be times when you have no choice but to eat UPF bread or, if you have kids, watch them eat it. It's okay. You are doing your best!

Other types of bread

As well as your sliced loaf, there are numerous other types of bread that will almost certainly catch you out if you are trying to quit UPF, such as:

- pitta bread;
- wraps;
- bagels;
- ciabattas;
- focaccias;
- crumpets;
- teacakes;
- paninis.

I'm sorry to have to break this news, but all of the above are filled with UPF – again, this is why they all look the same and last about a decade in your bread bin – and should be avoided. What you choose to do with this news is up to you. In my house we have mostly stopped buying them, although as wraps are a real staple of very popular family fajita nights, I've experimented with making them. They turned out okay, but don't have that plasticity of the shop variety (presumably because they don't contain any UPF!), so tend to snap and fall apart a bit when folded around the food. They taste lovely, though!

WRAPS

250g plain flour
Good grind of salt
2 tablespoons oil (olive, sunflower, vegetable, up to you)

Combine the flour and salt with the oil and knead into a dough. Split into about six to eight balls and roll out with a rolling pin, as thin as possible, but this time, you dry fry them in a large frying pan over a medium heat for one to two minutes each side, until golden and toasted. A bit like pancakes! Pretty easy.

Evening meals

I don't think you can replicate your old UPF evening menu when cooking from scratch, unless you are highly skilled and both time- and cash-rich. For example, if you were used to options like ready-made pies, curries with jar sauces, fishcakes, quiches, garlic bread and pizza, breaded and battered fish or chicken Kiev, you might find these a bit complicated to make. To make a pie, for example, means you've got to make pastry, the filling, get it all together and get it in the oven. I'm not saying it's impossible, but if you're not used to cooking or are lacking in confidence, it might be a bridge too far to start with. So my advice would be to simplify everything, then build up your skills and your repertoire gradually. Think about some of the simple, whole-ingredient meals you can make (there's a short list on page 259), meat or fish or eggs, served with vegetables or salad, and potatoes, rice or pasta. Start simple and then branch out by trying new recipes (see Resources, page 309).

A can of tomatoes
You can do so much with a can of tomatoes. Make sure you always have some in your cupboard. You absolutely don't need to buy jars of UPF tomato-based sauce – just use canned tomatoes. For a quick and easy supper, add a can of chopped tomatoes to a pan, a tin of drained tuna, salt, pepper, a pinch of chilli flakes, and a handful of black olives. Just heating it up is enough, then leave it to reduce for a few minutes if you can. You can also pimp it with onion (fried first in the saucepan before you add the tomatoes), chopped red pepper or chopped celery, chopped anchovy, fresh garlic or herbs, drained tinned chickpeas, butter beans or cannellini beans, a dash of Worcestershire sauce, smoked paprika or whatever else you feel might work well! But if you're really in a hurry, just a can

of tomatoes with a bit of seasoning, heated up and reduced slightly, with pasta stirred in and a good handful of cheese on top is better – and way cheaper – than that jar of UPF. You can also use tinned tomatoes in a huge variety of dishes from Bolognese to curry to soup, and as a basic tomato sauce on homemade pizza. Never leave the supermarket without canned tomatoes!

Pizza nights

This is a great way to have a UPF-free evening that the whole family will enjoy, and it's really not as hard as you might think. Obviously, you can buy ready-made pizza dough, pizza bases and even pizza dough 'mix', and although many contain palm and other oils, preservatives and even gums, if you look at the ingredients you can find some that are low or no UPF. But for a Saturday night family activity, making your own pizza dough is actually super easy. This recipe doesn't even require any proving (leaving to rise), and makes about four to six pizzas the size of a baking tray, depending on how thinly you roll it. If you are catering for fewer people, you can freeze whatever dough you don't need and use it another time.

PIZZA

For the dough
400g plain flour – doesn't have to be any special kind of flour, even the cheapest 'value' flour works just fine
7g sachet fast-action dried yeast
1 teaspoon salt

1 teaspoon caster sugar (leave this out, if you prefer)
2 tablespoons olive oil
225ml water

For the topping
1 × 400g tin tomatoes or 500g carton passata
1 × 200g ball mozzarella
300g grated cheese
And whatever else you like on a pizza!

Line a baking tray with baking paper. Put all the dry ingredients in a mixing bowl, and stir them around. Combine the oil and water in a jug and pour over the dry ingredients. Mix it around with your hands until you get a rough ball of dough. Then put a sprinkling of flour on a clean work surface and give it a quick knead until it feels a bit smoother.

Break the dough up into four to six balls, roughly the same size, and use a rolling pin to roll it out to about the size of a standard baking tray (approx. 32×23 cm). This will give you four to six pizzas. Use plenty of sprinklings of flour to stop it sticking to your surface or the rolling pin. Try and get it as thin as you can. Once you've rolled it out, you might have to fold it in half and then in half again to gently transport it to your baking tray, and then 'unfold' it in situ.

Then the fun bit starts! If you want to keep it really simple, you can just use passata or even a tin of chopped tomatoes for your tomato sauce. Or you can make your own by reducing chopped tomatoes or passata in a pan with garlic, herbs, etc. As we're in the business of making a non-UPF life easy here,

I'm going to tell you not to bother – just chuck on the tomatoes, straight from the tin. I won't tell anyone if you don't.

Spread out a thin layer of passata or chopped tomatoes on your dough. Then everyone can add their own toppings of choice: grated Cheddar, mozzarella, pepperoni, olives, anchovies, tuna, thinly sliced bell pepper, sliced fresh tomatoes, thinly sliced mushroom, ham, tinned pineapple, capers, cooked chicken, fresh chilli...well, you know what you like on your own pizza! If anyone likes 'stuffed crust' you can do that too, just put a little line of cheese around the edge before you put the tomato on, and sort of fold it over and squish it together – another job kids will love, if you have them about the house. Then into an oven, preheated to 200°C/180°C fan/gas 6, they go. They take about 10–15 mins, depending on how you like your pizza, so just keep an eye on them. Once cooked, you can add fresh rocket or chopped parsley, chilli flakes, salt, pepper, etc. You will never eat frozen pizza again!

PIZZA PASTA

If you haven't got the bandwidth for pizza dough, this is a recipe I invented and that my kids absolutely adore. It's basically a pasta bake, with a bit of up-selling involved.

1 onion, chopped
2 garlic cloves, chopped
1 carrot, peeled and sliced
1 stick of celery, chopped
1 red bell pepper, chopped and deseeded

2 × 400g tins tomatoes
500g dried pasta shapes, e.g. fusilli
1 × 200g mozzarella ball
Salt, pepper, chilli powder
150g Cheddar cheese
1 packet pepperoni (see page 294)

In a large saucepan fry the onion for about five minutes on a medium heat until soft. Add the garlic and fry for one more minute. Then add the carrot, celery, and red pepper. Stir for another minute then add both tins of tomatoes, along with salt and pepper to taste and a pinch of chilli powder. Leave on a low to medium heat, stirring occasionally, for about 30 minutes. About halfway through that time, cook and drain the pasta and pre-heat the oven to 200°C/180°C fan/gas 6. When all the vegetables in the pan are soft, use a stick blender to whizz up your sauce until blended. Add in the pasta and mix well, then transfer to a large oven-proof dish. Sprinkle the grated Cheddar on the top, and tear up the mozzarella and dot it around the Cheddar. Lay the slices of pepperoni on the top and bake in the oven for about 15 minutes, or until the cheese is bubbling and beginning to brown. Serve with salad if you wish, but relax knowing there is a lot of veg in the sauce! This serves roughly six people. Variations: use different pizza toppings instead: replace pepperoni with thinly sliced mushroom, ham and pineapple, black olives, torn chicken, or whatever you wish. For a vegan version leave out the cheese. And in all cases, be sure to sing, 'When the moon hits your eye like a big pizza pie, that's AMORE!', when serving it up!

Bringing FLAVOUR

Almost all of us are used to the UPF flavours that can pack a punch, whether that's smoky bacon crisps or jars of curry sauce. So one part of your quitting/reducing UPF adventure is learning how to deliver big taste so that food never gets boring. It's better to learn how to season and flavour food yourself, because otherwise you stray into the danger zone of rogue UPF ingredients. For example, if you are buying meat and it says 'honey glazed' or 'BBQ ribs', etc., check the ingredients. You might find that it's not just honey or BBQ seasoning, and that your meat has been coated in other ingredients too. Similarly, some of the sachets of seasoning (for example, packets in 'fajita kits' or ready-made meat rubs) you can buy can contain UPF ingredients as well as just the spices you are looking for. I recommend stocking up on a few basic seasonings and spices:

- salt and pepper (freshly ground is best, so get salt and pepper mills if you can and buy coarse sea salt and peppercorns);
- chilli (powdered or flakes);
- ground cumin;
- paprika / smoked paprika;
- dried thyme, oregano or marjoram (all fairly similar, so just one will do if on a budget);
- garlic (fresh is great but fiddly if you are short on time, so get some powdered rather than the purée, which can sometimes have preservatives. Check the label!).

As you get more adventurous, you might like to try cooking with fresh garlic, chillies and ginger or fresh herbs (you can grow some of these if you have a garden or space for some small pots):

- coriander / cilantro (great in salads and curries);
- parsley (goes with almost every dish);
- rosemary;
- thyme;
- sage;
- bay leaves (you can buy these dried as well).

HOMEMADE POTATO WEDGES

several potatoes
oil (enough to coat)
salt and pepper
spices: paprika, cumin, chilli, oregano (optional)
garlic cloves, peeled and halved (optional)
garlic powder (optional)

Get a bag of potatoes and chop them, skin on, into chunks or wedges around the size of your thumb. Allow about two medium-sized potatoes per person. Chuck them in your roasting tin and splosh on some oil – and this is when you can experiment with flavour. You could go for plain and simply grind on a generous bit of salt and pepper. Or you could sprinkle over a teaspoon of paprika. Perhaps try a mix: paprika, cumin, chilli (if you like it hot), and oregano. Add some whole cloves of garlic, just take them off the bulb, peel them, chop them in half and nestle them in among your spuds, or a sprinkle of garlic powder. Make sure you toss the potatoes around in the oil and spices so they are evenly coated, then put in a pre-heated oven on around 200°C/180°C fan/gas 6 for 20–30 minutes. You will never make UPF oven chips again!

Condiments

Ketchup, BBQ sauce, HP sauce, mayo, salad dressing, chilli sauce, mustard – these dinner-table staples are a mixed bag. This is one of those areas where, now that you've had the UPF lightbulb switched on, you're going to have to do your own thinking about which condiments matter to you and how UPF-filled your favourite brands are. The good news, especially if you have kids, is that most of the main brands of ketchup are okay, and if you don't trust what they mean when they use the generic and rather vague term 'spice', then there are organic varieties available that are even better. Mayonnaise, on the other hand (which I live and die for), contains something called EDTA (see page 31). You can buy more expensive artisan-type brands that are EDTA-free, or you can make your own.

EASY MAYO

1 egg
1 tablespoon white or red wine vinegar
1 tablespoon Dijon mustard
Pinch of salt
240ml oil

Add the egg, vinegar, mustard and salt to a jug and then using a stick blender give it a quick whizz. Slowly add the oil and keep whizzing it as you pour. It should emulsify and come together fairly easily. This makes one small jar, which will keep in the fridge for two days.

Other condiments vary. The leading brand of English mustard contains xanthan gum and is ranked as UPF by the Open Food Facts app, and the leading Dijon contains potassium metabisulphite, ranking it as 'processed'. HP sauce, also known as 'brown sauce', is usually okay. Lots of shop-bought salad dressings contain gums and emulsifiers, as do spicy peri-peri-type sauces, and some spicy relishes and hot sauces like sriracha can also contain a thickener called 'modified maize starch'. Your best bet is to either investigate the practicalities of making your own, or have a look around, either online or in the more expensive supermarkets, for more 'artisanal' or organic brands that have fewer nasties.

When I worked for the Dumas family in France (see page 51), they taught me to make a salad dressing that they poured over literally everything, and I've been making it ever since.

THE DUMAS DRESSING

Okay, so all you have to remember about this dressing is the ratio 1:1:3. You can make it straight into the salad bowl, and then pile your salad on top, tossing it in the dressing when you're ready to serve. Put it into the bowl in this order.

1 tablespoon Dijon mustard
1 tablespoon red wine vinegar
3 tablespoons sunflower oil

This was the way the Dumas family taught it to me, but you can use a different vinegar if you like, and olive oil if you prefer. With your 1:1:3 formula, you can scale it up or down in quantity, just keep your ratios roughly the same. It takes a minute or two of mixing with a fork or a miniature whisk to get it to all come together and emulsify. When it does, it will be a smooth, uniform, creamy texture, with no oily patches or lumps.

Monsieur Dumas used to extol the virtues of sunflower oil – 'how wonderful,' he said, 'that it came from such a beautiful flower.' But since I've been researching UPF, I've realized that not everyone feels this way, which brings us to the question of seed oils.

Oils

If you join any of the large Facebook groups where UPF is discussed, you are sure to find people fighting each other about seed oils. So, at the risk of getting myself cancelled (again), I'm here to tell you that SEED OILS ARE NOT UPF – at least, not according to the Nova classification (see page 20), which puts all oils as Nova Group 2 – 'processed culinary ingredients'.

Examples of seed oils:
- rapeseed / canola oil;
- vegetable oil (most often made with rapeseed);
- soybean oil;
- sunflower oil;
- cottonseed oil;
- safflower oil;
- rice bran oil;
- grapeseed oil;
- corn oil;
- sesame oil;
- palm kernel oil.

So why the concern? Firstly, the way in which many seed oils are produced, which involves a highly industrialized process of refinement, bleaching and extraction via solvents, sounds an awful lot like 'ultra-processing' to some. Secondly, from a health point of view, seed oils contain an omega-6 fatty acid called linoleic acid that has been linked to inflammation. This is true of seed oils even if they are 'cold-pressed' – so while buying, say, cold-pressed sunflower oil solves your chemical refinement fears, it's still just as high in omega-6 as the cheaper stuff.

The problem with omega-6 is that we need it in small quantities, but the Western diet currently contains too much of it. We are supposed to eat roughly equal amounts of omega-6 and omega-3, but it's currently estimated that we are eating more like sixteen times the amount of omega-6 than omega-3. This, say some, is leading to inflammation and other health problems, although others dispute this theory, with some arguing that omega-6 is good for us, as long as we balance it out with enough omega-3. This could be where the problem lies because, with a diet high in UPF, we're unlikely to be getting that balance right.

It's worth remembering, though, that these increased levels of seed oil consumption are coming from the foods we eat, not the oils we choose to use for frying or making salad dressing. Once you start checking ingredients lists to see if they are UPF, you're going to suddenly notice just how many foods contain seed oils. For example: dairy-free milks, oven chips, ready-made pies and sausage rolls, various breads, such as part-baked rolls and pittas – seed oils are in so many products. If we are eating all of these products, and also not eating much oily fish for omega-3, then there's definitely an argument that this isn't the diet we have evolved to eat.

The problem with vilifying seed oils is that the alternatives, in particular extra virgin olive oil, are more expensive. With all food, a good general rule is: eat the best you can afford. If, for you, that means frying your breakfast eggs in vegetable oil or using sunflower oil in the Dumas dressing, that's a brilliant step up from having a bowl of sugary cereal or a supermarket sandwich. You are not eating a bellyful of UPF, and this is a brilliant thing.

So to recap:

- No oils are UPF according to Nova, but some cheaper oils are made by a highly industrialized process and you might prefer to avoid these oils.
- To avoid industrially processed oils, choose 'cold-pressed' oils of any variety, and/or extra virgin olive oil.
- Seed oils, however they are produced, concern some people because of the higher levels of omega-6 they contain. But if you are only using them sparingly in cooking, rather than eating large quantities of them in UPF, then this is probably fine, especially if you are taking care of your omega-3 consumption by eating oily fish once or twice a week.

Butter

I've tried to be as even-handed as possible in this book, but I'm now going to go out on a limb and say: STOP EATING ANY KIND OF SPREAD THAT ISN'T BUTTER. Yes, even that posh 'spreadable' butter you've been getting. IT'S NOT BUTTER. Well, technically it's 40 per cent butter, but the rest of it is…guess what? Seed oils! Even the fancy one that says it's made with olive oil also contains rapeseed oil and palm oil, plus two different emulsifiers and 'flavourings'. Please stop eating this revolting stuff, get it out of your fridge, and eat butter instead. Margarine, baking spread, spreadable butter, soft spread, buttery spread…all of it, it's ALL UPF. Chuck it in the bin. Eat butter.

Vegan and 'free from'

As I have one child with a severe dairy and egg allergy, I am no stranger to vegan and 'free from' products. And yes, they are all UPF as well. The 'vegan' spreads are all UPF, and most of the dairy-free 'milks' are too. So are the vegan 'ice creams', biscuits, chocolate bars, yoghurts (yes, even the 'natural' or 'plain' vegan yoghurt is UPF), puddings, and cakes. Worse still are the vegan 'cheeses' and pretend 'meats', which are all chock-full of emulsifiers, gums, preservatives, and long lists of ingredients that simply are *not food*. The most shocking thing about these products is the way they have been sold to people as a healthy option with the slogan 'plant-based'. If I handed you a glass filled with rapeseed oil, modified starch, dried rice syrup, agar gelling agent and xanthan gum, would you drink it? Go on, it's PLANT-BASED!!

This 'plant-based' idea has been co-opted from the world of nutrition, which is quite rightly recommending our diets be based around as many plants as possible (you know, the ones that still look like actual plants and haven't been industrially pulverized into weird concoctions yet). Slapping 'PLANT-BASED' on the packaging of as many UPF products as they can get away with is a form of advertising hypnosis. It's a technique known as 'anchoring', in which we are encouraged to build an association between the phrase 'plant-based' and ideas of healthy, natural, wholesome nutrition, with a little bit of saving the planet thrown in for good measure. Eventually, we just need to see this phrase for it to trigger a positive response, and into the trolley goes our wholesome 'plant-based' product. Well, I'm here to clap my hands loudly in front of your face and tell you, 'you're back in the room'. Stop buying these UPF products.

If you want to have a 'plant-based' diet for health or environmental reasons, please do so, but there is absolutely no need to incorporate the fake UPF cheeses and meats into that diet. Researchers at Imperial College London recently found that eating these 'plant-based' UPFs can increase your risk of cardiovascular disease by as much as 7 per cent, whilst cutting them out and replacing them with *actual plants* can reduce your risk by the same amount.[2] Going 'vegan' is in itself a complex topic of dietary health, so if you are doing this, do seek nutritional advice.

If, like my family, your reason for choosing 'free from' is not veganism but allergies, then you can get some 'plant-based' milks that are not UPF – unfortunately, these often tend to be the more expensive, organic brands – but I did recently discover that the budget 'Everyday Essentials' soya milk in Aldi is just water, hulled soya beans and sea salt – and it's incredibly cheap. You can also make your own milk substitutes, and then make these into your own vegan 'butter' – there are various recipes online. If you are going for shop-bought 'free from' products, check labels and think about whether the product is really needed, would be my best advice.

Bacon, chorizo, cured meats, ham, pepperoni, salami, saucisson

Frankly, this could be a wish-list for me if I was going to be stranded on a desert island and could only take one type of food. I was alarmed, therefore, to discover people were talking about some of these items in the context of UPF and, bacon butty in hand, decided to investigate further. The problem that people seem to have with cured meats is that they have been linked to cancer, and it's suggested that this could be because they contain nitrites and nitrates. However, it would be wrong to suggest they are UPF. They are 'processed', but not 'ultra-processed'. If you're quitting UPF, you can still eat these items (phew!), but the current NHS advice is to limit red and processed meats to 70g or less a day. If you so wish, you can seek out versions 'made without nitrites' but, confusingly, these more expensive items are cured with celery juice, which is also high in natural nitrates. It's a bit of a minefield, but the key point is that these foods are not generally UPF, therefore can be enjoyed as part of a balanced diet high in plants.

Sausages, on the other hand – by which I mean good old British bangers – are much more likely to be UPF, containing a variety of gums, emulsifiers and preservatives. If you really love sausages, have a look at the ingredients and pick the one with the fewest additives, try your local butcher to see what they put in theirs, or just limit them to an occasional treat. Other types of speciality sausage and meat products, like black pudding and haggis, tend to be UPF-free, but check labels.

What's for dessert?

The whole concept of having a sweet course at the end of a meal is a modern invention and arguably one that we could do without. However, as leaving it there is likely to make me very unpopular with the sweet-toothed among you, let's just say that if you want to quit UPF, you can definitely kiss goodbye to most supermarket puddings, cakes and desserts. Ice cream has already got a mention, although you can find UPF-free vanilla – check the ingredients list. Say no to flavoured yoghurts, and please also stop eating shop-bought chocolate mousse, microwave steamed puddings, custard, jelly, fruit pie, cheesecake, trifle...the lot of it! Not only is it full of sugar, it's also ultra-processed and full of gums, oils, syrups, emulsifiers and stabilisers. Don't put it in the trolley – your body will thank you. If you do feel the need for a sweet food after a meal, you could try:

- natural yoghurt with fruit and honey;
- peeled, frozen bananas, blended, make a sort of 'ice cream', and you could try adding peanut butter;
- frozen fruit (bought in bags) can also be blended with a little water and a dash of honey to make 'sorbet';
- homemade ice cream (invest in an ice cream-maker or try various online recipes that don't require one);
- baked apples (core an apple, place on a baking tray and fill the centre with a mix of raisins/sultanas, sugar and cinnamon, and a knob of butter, bake for 20 minutes);
- pancakes with lemon and sugar (see recipe page 264);
- an apple and a thick slice of good Cheddar (a favourite of my Canadian dad, who also always ate his apple pie with cheese rather than cream);
- fruit crumble (probably one of the easiest homemade puddings, the topping is just butter and flour gently rubbed together with a sprinkle of sugar on top – there are recipes online).

Soft drinks

There have probably been enough mentions in this book of the evidence against fizzy drinks/sodas for you to know that it's best to cut these out. There might be an argument for keeping other UPF items in your diet, but I really can't think of a single one for cola – we just don't need it and it's incredibly bad for us. Water, tea, coffee, herbal teas – these are all fine, but not soda. Squash is also usually UPF, although some of the posher, organic 'cordials' are often okay. Most so-called 'sports' and 'energy' drinks are absolutely 100 per cent UPF, as are 'protein shakes'. During the writing this book I chose a supermarket iced coffee, only to discover it contained not just coffee and milk as I had imagined, but two different gums and a whole load of other nasties. Drinks marketed towards kids are also usually packed with additives. Once you start thinking about it and reading the ingredients, you really do wonder why we are all putting these ingredients into our and our children's bodies, when water is so readily available. Definitely time for a change. Try adding slices of lemon, cucumber, orange, lime, or a handful of frozen berries to a jug of iced water instead, or, if everyone is missing squash, a very small amount of fruit juice topped up with water. Fruit juice itself is not a UPF, and nor are most fruit smoothies, but it's not recommended to drink too much of either of these as they can cause blood sugar spikes, and they don't have the same benefits as eating whole fruits because most of the fibre has been broken down (think of the food matrix, see page 46).

Alcoholic drinks

Without getting into the ins and outs of the benefits and drawbacks of alcohol to health (most of the world's Blue Zones drink it, but they do so with food and not to excess), let's just say that wine (both red and white) and beer are not UPF. Where you get into UPF territory is with flavoured spirits, cocktails in a can, some fruity ciders, and 'alcopops'. Obviously, if you use fizzy drinks as mixers, then they are UPF (see previous page), and although whisky, gin and vodka are technically categorized as Nova 4 and therefore ultra-processed, this seems to be a bit of anomaly and the mixer is more likely to be truly UPF in the sense of nasty additives, etc. If you want to drink at all, you are better off with a wine or beer, it seems, and probably better still with an organic wine or an artisan beer. Perhaps the rule of 'everything in moderation' could come in useful here, especially on a hot summer's day when a jug of Pimm's and lemonade is on offer!

Takeaways and eating out

This is another mixed bag that you'll need to navigate as best as you can. Larger chain restaurants and takeaway services can often use bought-in sauces and frozen preparations that are high in UPF. On a menu, look for the options that are more 'wholefood' based, like salads or meat/fish and two veg. You can always ask for a list of ingredients and any good restaurant should be happy to provide them. Some people do find that once they have stopped eating so much UPF, if they do have fast-food or a UPF takeaway, they feel almost a 'hangover' from it, as if their body rejects it more than it used to. If you absolutely love curry or Chinese food as a treat, and you know your local haunt is using a lot of UPF, it might be worth searching for your favourite dish online and having a go at making it yourself. Although the spices may be an initial investment, once you are set up you will find that the results are absolutely delicious. Think of it as a whole new hobby!

Batch-cooking

If you want to go UPF-free, batch-cooking is your new best friend – providing you have a freezer. It can save you money, too, as you will probably use less gas or electric and have less food waste. The entry level to batch-cooking simply means that every time you cook something suitable, you make at least double what you will need and freeze the rest. So if you're making Bolognese, or soup, or stew, you just portion up and bag 50 per cent of what you've cooked. Some people go up another level and set aside time at the weekend to do a really big batch-cooking session, where they not only prepare meals for the freezer, they also cook 'base recipes', for example mince and tomatoes, that can be defrosted and transformed quickly into different dishes, such as a pasta sauce, a chilli or a cottage pie. And for the ultimate in batch-cooking, you can even get together for batch-cooking clubs or parties, where each person cooks a dish and everybody then takes away some portions of everyone else's creations. Batch-cooking is brilliant for families but it's equally useful if you live on your own, because it can be hard to be motivated to cook from scratch every night if it's just for yourself. You'll need to clear some freezer space – but that shouldn't be difficult once you stop buying all those UPF ice creams and pizzas!

Not sweating the small stuff

Everyone will find their own approach to UPF, just as we all do with everything else. Some people want to completely get rid of every trace of it, while others make small changes, or opt for an 80/20 approach. There is no one right way and as we live in a culture where often UPF is the easiest, quickest, most normalized and most accessible option, I would urge you to go easy on yourself. You might not be able to go completely UPF-free, but there are quick, high-impact changes you can make. Ditch the breakfast cereal, ice cream, fizzy drinks, snack bars and crisps, and change your approach to bread. This will automatically take you to an entirely new place in terms of your diet.

As you make spaces in your day by removing these major sources of UPF, you will find that you begin to fill them instead with wholefoods, which will be doing you all kinds of good. Pat yourself on the back for this. And please be wary of becoming too obsessed with a purist approach to your diet, perhaps fuelled by internet chat rooms and Facebook groups, which are often set up under the umbrella of discussing UPF but then depart down a variety of rabbit holes. It's definitely not healthy to be stressed and anxious about everything you eat, and the fact that you are reading this book shows that you already care very much about yourself, your health, and the health of your nearest and dearest. Also, please don't beat yourself up about choices you have made in the past that cannot be changed. Today is the first day of a new start, and a chance for you to develop a relationship with food preparation, eating, and sharing food with others that is positive and exciting. Don't let the impossibility of perfection spoil that adventure for you. Keep going. Stir the pot. Lick the spoon. And don't sweat the small stuff.

Postscript: A dog's dinner

Although this book is here to ask the question, *'but what about women?'*, I was led to write it, at least in part, by an interaction with my dog, a seven-year-old Jack Russell who goes by the name of Cookie. For her entire life I've been feeding Cookie from a tin or a bag clearly marked DOG FOOD, and for her part she has been gulping it down without question – until one day, about two years ago. *Pop* – I opened the tin as usual, forked the mushy brown stuff into a dish and placed it on the floor before her. And then, there was a moment. She looked at the food, and she looked at me, and I looked at her, and it was as if we both had the same thought: 'that really does look flipping disgusting.' Turning her attention back to the bowl, she seemed to give a little sigh of resignation, and then, somewhat more reluctantly than usual, she ate it. Well, she is a dog, after all.

Our little inter-species interaction started me thinking, though, about the stuff on the plates of both humans and dogs and the nutritional responsibility we willingly hand over to food companies. Just as fish cannot see the water in which they swim, UPF surrounds us completely and has done for most or all of our lives. It's so close to our eyeballs, we just don't notice it anymore; it is, simply, 'what we eat'. *Pop* – we open the tin labelled 'FOOD'. We don't question. Hopefully this book has opened your eyes and made you ask, just as Cookie and I did that day, 'hang on, what actually IS this stuff?' Once you've had that thought, you can't unthink it. Change begins the moment we realize the problem is right there in front of us, staring us square in the face.

After the lightbulb moment, however, the rest of the process of change is often more complex and difficult. Firstly, it requires forgiveness: for past errors, and also for the errors we are bound to make as we take the next, hesitant steps. A few decades of ultra-processed food has deskilled us; many of us lack the knowledge or the confidence to prepare food from scratch, daily. The experimental phase of not-quite-knowing-what-you're-doing is inevitably expensive, because corner-cutting and economizing take time to learn. There will be days when we manage without UPF and days when we fall back on the old ways. *Pop* – we open the tin. On those days, we must forgive ourselves, and try again the next day. We mustn't give up. All progress is two steps forward and one step back. The idea that you have an epiphany and then do everything perfectly from that moment onwards is an unhelpful myth.

But change we must. Once you begin to think differently about food, you can't go back. For me, writing this book has forever altered the way I look at each packet and tin; I stop and ask, 'what actually IS this stuff?' And when I think about my physical and mental health, I always now consider what I've been eating as a piece of the puzzle, especially if I'm feeling less than optimal. I think more about my microbes, too, and how I might feed these little friends, in particular that Sea Witch (remember page 124), with fibre or a big dollop of kimchi. It's made me want to try even harder with my kids' diets, and to give them skills in the kitchen and a passion for good food that will stay with them long after they fly the nest. And as I approach my fifties, it's encouraged me to pay more attention to the food I eat as a way of hopefully maximizing my chances of a healthier second half of life, in just the same way I was already doing in terms of strength training and fitness. Making time to prepare and eat good food, rather like making time to exercise, can sometimes be fun and appealing, and can sometimes be a chore – but either way, it's worth trying your best to make a habit of it.

Beyond the personal, writing this book has opened my eyes to the bigger picture. In a position of privilege, with the funds to buy decent food, a warm house to cook it in, and the time and know-how to do so (yes, I even have time to worry about the quality of food my dog is eating), I know that people like me making change at an individual level simply isn't enough. Even with all the resources at my disposal, I have found it hard enough to reduce my UPF intake; people with less skill, time, or income than me are going to need help and support with this. We need corporations, politicians and policy-makers to turn this situation around, enforcing change through legislation, education, funding and strong leadership. At times, particularly when researching the environment chapter, I have felt that the picture is bleak. I feel a deep, existential worry that we have abandoned Mother Nature in our pursuit of unlimited possessions and monetary wealth and that there are not enough people in positions of power who are bothered enough by this to effect change. Our problem with ultra-processed food is just one slice of a rather dystopian pie that represents our current and unprecedented drift away from interconnectedness – with each other and with our natural environment. Every plastic packet and bag of UPF, piled high and often wasted, seems to represent our world of extremes in which many go hungry while a select few have more than they could ever need. We count ourselves lucky to live in a time of such abundance, where we can think of a product in bed at 11 p.m. and it can arrive at our house the next morning; where we can fill our trollies knowing – but not really minding – that at least some of the food we buy won't make it out of the packaging but will instead go straight from fridge to bin. But it's time to stop thinking of this as 'lucky' and start asking more questions about our direction of travel. We don't just have enough, we have too much. As well as demanding change at policy level, we also all need to have a complete mindset shift and start to value quality over quantity again.

And so, what about women? For most of recorded history, women have been prevented from having a casting vote – often literally. It is overwhelmingly men who have shaped our current world and decided our values. Looking around, I can see plenty of their achievements, but boy-oh-boy is there room for improvement. As women who now have a voice, we must demand change. The current ways are destructive and unsustainable. As we watch the thankless exploitation of the environment, we must say: *enough*. As we see profit being prioritized over our health, we can vote with our wallets. UPF has co-opted women's desire for freedom and dished us up the fake version in a tin marked 'food'. But it is not feeding us, it is making us sick, and we need to stop buying it. Every purchase of UPF maintains this business model, this status quo. Conversely, every home-cooked meal, rather than being a submission to patriarchy as we've been told, is in fact a radical act of resistance. 'Going back to the kitchen' is a notion we can all – whether male or female – reclaim as progressive, rather than regressive. It's a chance to be resourceful, to nurture ourselves and others, to bring flavour and human connection; it is as vital for our health and wellbeing as exercise, nature and creativity; it is as vital for the planet as reducing, reusing and recycling. Simple meals of whole-foods are in fact a statement piece and they say: *there is a better way, change is possible, and I'm not giving up.*

Since Cookie looked sideways that day at the mush in her bowl, I've discovered that UPF companies make dog food, too – Mars make Pedigree, for example, and PURINA is made by Nestlé. After a lifetime of mindlessly opening a tin, I'm now trying to work out what dogs are actually supposed to eat. Just like making the switch away from UPF for humans, this is a journey fraught with pitfalls and setbacks, with online searches turning up pages written by pet-food companies and Facebook groups full of misinformation, one-upmanship and in-fighting. Sometimes, it's overwhelming, and I find myself dishing up the factory-formed kibble. But today I'm cooking up a storm – *tripes de boeuf vertes avec cou de dinde* – in other words, cow stomach and turkey neck. It absolutely stinks, but Cookie seems to like it very much. If she could talk, I think she'd say it beats that muck in the tin by a country mile. In fact, I swear I heard her mutter contentedly the other day, as she lay on the sofa in a post-prandial haze, 'finally. Some actual FOOD.'

Acknowledgements

I'm hugely grateful to the myriad of people who played a role in the creation of this book. First and foremost, I would like to thank my partner George and my children Bess, Ursula and Albie, who cheered me on with this project from the very start, and, towards the end, even went on holiday without me so that I could get it finished. I would not be who I am without these four very special humans.

To my kids, I'm really sorry that I've basically ruined super noodles for you, but I respect you for ploughing ahead and eating them anyway. I'd also like to thank my mum, Pauline Hill, who is always there for me, cheering me on. Thanks also to my dad, no longer here, but one of the trio to whom this book is dedicated – I wish he and my grandad Bert (he of the cheese wire) could see me getting my fourth book out into the world. They would no doubt burst with pride.

Friends are also a writer's champions. Thanks in particular to Anna Wharton, who has become a dear friend over the course of the writing of this book, which led to her eventually providing me with a new love of my life, Polly the Labrador puppy. Other amazing humans who always have my back include my oldest friends Erika and Will, my neighbours Kirsten and Richard, Sharon, Emma B, and so many others. Then there are the many online groups and individuals who support me – the writers' WhatsApp groups, the feminist Facebook groups, the women who come to my Substack writing group, to name just a few.

Many, many experts responded to my cries for help during the writing process. Rather than try to write an exhaustive list and risk almost certainly leaving someone out, let me just say a particular thanks to Rob Percival at the Soil Association and Carlos Monteiro and his team, and beyond that, to anyone quoted within these pages, and to those who simply patiently explained their research – I am forever grateful.

Last but not least, heartfelt thanks to Jane at Graham Maw Christie, who is always calm and steadfast, and to the team at HQ – Danielle, Rachael, Lisa, Rachel, Kathy, Kom, Tamsin – and anyone else who helped.

And to you, the reader – thank you too. This book would be a fairly pointless activity without you! Enjoy your journey back to human connection: it all starts with food.

RESOURCES

Apps

Open Food Facts: check if your food is UPF by scanning the barcode
https://world.openfoodfacts.org/

Yuka: get a rating and ingredients for your toiletries and cosmetics by scanning the barcode
https://yuka.io/en/

Campaign groups

Sustain: an alliance for better food and farming
https://www.sustainweb.org/

Sustain runs several campaigns, including:
The Children's Food Campaign
https://www.sustainweb.org/childrens-food-campaign/

Real Bread Campaign
https://www.sustainweb.org/realbread/
Campaign for Better Hospital Food
https://www.sustainweb.org/hospitalfood/

The Soil Association: a charity focused on the effect of agriculture on the environment
https://www.soilassociation.org/
Women's Environmental Network: connecting women, health, equity and environmental justice
https://www.wen.org.uk/
Bite Back: youth activism for a better food system
https://www.biteback2030.com/
Women's Voices for the Earth: envisioning a world free from toxic chemicals
https://womensvoices.org/
Farmers Against Farmwashing: campaigning against misleading marketing by supermarkets
https://stopfarmwashing.co.uk/
The Food Foundation: campaigning for a sustainable food system
https://foodfoundation.org.uk/
includes the campaign **Children's Right2Food**
https://foodfoundation.org.uk/initiatives/childrens-right2food
Food, Farming and Countryside Commission: helping shape the future of food and farming, including a Citizen Manifesto
https://fcc.co.uk/our-people/commissioners

Baby Milk Action: campaigning against misleading marketing by the baby-food industry
https://www.babymilkaction.org/

Migrateful: cookery classes taught by refugees and migrants
https://www.migrateful.org/

Women in the Food Industry: championing women in the UK food industry
https://womeninthefoodindustry.com/

First Steps Nutrition: supporting eating well from preconception to five years
https://www.firststepsnutrition.org/

Recipe websites

https://www.bbcgoodfood.com/
https://www.bbc.co.uk/food
https://www.epicurious.com/
https://www.allrecipes.com/

Books to read next

About UPF:

Ultra-Processed People: The Science Behind Food that Isn't Food by Chris van Tulleken

Unprocessed: What Your Diet is Doing to Your Brain by Kimberley Wilson – how the food we eat is fuelling our mental health crisis

Metabolical: The Lure and the Lies of Processed Food, Nutrition, and Modern Medicine by Dr Robert H. Lustig – the truth about processed food and how it poisons people and the planet

Wider thinking:

Braiding Sweetgrass: Indigenous Wisdom, Scientific Knowledge and the Teaching of Plants by Robin Wall Kimmerer
Regenesis: Feeding the World without Devouring the Planet by George Monbiot
The Wilderness Cure: Ancient Wisdom in a Modern World by Mo Wilde
The Omnivore's Dilemma: A Natural History of Four Meals by Michael Pollan

Cookbooks:

(There are SO many! These three are a good starting point for ease and cost.)

The Roasting Tin by Rukmini Iyer – a series of books, all of them 'one dish dinners' / traybakes
The Batch Lady: Shop Once, Cook Once, Eat Well All Week by Suzanne Mulholland – the definitive guide to batch cooking (and by the same author: *The Batch Lady: Cooking on a Budget*)

RESOURCES

Feed your Family For £20 a Week: 100 Budget-Friendly Batch-Cooking Recipes You'll All Enjoy by Lorna Cooper – cost-effective recipes designed to feed a family

Endnotes

Introduction: And what about women?

1. Pounis, George, et al., 'Reduction in menopause symptom severity following a personalised app-based dietary intervention program: a pre-post longitudinal analysis of the ZOE PREDICT 3 study', Nutrition Society Congress 2–5 July, 2024 (www.morressier.com/o/event/6655b1890ec964e1c ccef602/article/6671b57ac9b69e0de564d19e)
2. Samuthpongtorn, Chatpol, et al., 'Consumption of Ultra-processed Food and Risk of Depression', *JAMA Netw Open.* September 20, 2023;6(9):e2334770 (jamanetwork.com/ journals/jamanetworkopen/fullarticle/2809727)
3. Jacka, Felice N., et al., 'A randomised controlled trial of dietary improvement for adults with major depression', *BMC Medicine*, 28 December 2018 (pmc.ncbi.nlm.nih.gov/articles/ PMC5282719/)
4. Rossato, Sinara Laurini, et al., '501 Association between ultra-processed food intake with risk of systemic lupus erythematosus in women', *Cutaneous Lupus & Photosensitivity*, 16 May 2024 (lupus.bmj.com/content/11/ Suppl_2/A31.2)

5. Borland, Sophie, 'UK government's nutrition advisers are paid by world's largest food companies', *BMJ*, 11 September 2024 (www.bmj.com/content/386/bmj.q1909)
6. Valicente, Vinicius M., et al., 'Ultraprocessed Foods and Obesity Risk: A Critical Review of Reported Mechanisms', *Advances in Nutrition*, Vol 14, Issue 4, July 2023 (www.sciencedirect.com/science/article/pii/S2161831323002910)
7. May, Natasha and Ittimani, Luca, 'Australia's health star rating system exploited by companies making ultra-processed foods, experts say', *The Guardian*, 24 July 2024 (www.theguardian.com/australia-news/article/2024/jul/25/australias-health-star-rating-system-exploited-by-companies-making-ultra-processed-foods-experts-say)
8. Aubrey, Allison, 'Worldwide, women cook twice as much as men: One country bucks the trend', *NPR*, 30 October 2023 (www.npr.org/sections/health-shots/2023/10/30/1209473449/worldwide-women-cook-twice-as-much-as-men-one-country-bucks-the-trend)
9. Wakefield, Jane, 'People devote third of waking time to mobile apps', BBC News, 12 January 2022 (www.bbc.co.uk/news/technology-59952557)
10. Soil Association, 'The future of British farming outside the EU', (www.soilassociation.org/media/10560/soil-association-report.pdf), accessed September 2024

Chapter 1. So, what is ultra-processed food (UPF)?

1. Prescott, Susan L., et al., 'Not Food: Time to Call Ultra-Processed Products by Their True Name', *Gastronomy*, 8 April 2024 (www.mdpi.com/2813-513X/2/2/4#B24-gastronom)
2. Monteiro, Carlos A., 'Nutrition and health. The issue is not food, nor nutrients, so much as processing', Cambridge University Press, 1 May 2009 (www.cambridge.org/core/

journals/public-health-nutrition/article/nutrition-and-health-the-issue-is-not-food-nor-nutrients-so-much-asprocessing/0C514FC9DB264538F83D5D34A81BB10A), accessed September 2024
3. Open Food Facts, 'Nova groups for food processing' (world.openfoodfacts.org/nova), accessed September 2024
4. UK Flour Millers (www.ukflourmillers.org/statistics#), accessed September 2024
5. BBC News, 'Cadbury drops "glass and a half" phrase from wrappers', 28 September 2010 (www.bbc.com/news/business-11427357)

Chapter 2. What's the problem with UPF?

1. Hall, Kevin D., et al., 'Ultra-Processed Diets Cause Excess Calorie Intake and Weight Gain: An Inpatient Randomized Controlled Trial of Ad Libitum Food Intake', *Cell Metab*, 2 July 2019 (pubmed.ncbi.nlm.nih.gov/31105044/)
2. Lane, Melissa M., et al., 'Ultra-processed food exposure and adverse health outcomes: umbrella review of epidemiological meta-analyses', *BMJ*, 28 February 2024 (www.bmj.com/content/384/bmj-2023-077310)
3. Latif, Samreen, et al., 'Junk food consumption in relation to menstrual abnormalities among adolescent girls: A comparative cross sectional study', *Pakistan Journal of Medical Sciences,* November–December 2022 (pmc.ncbi.nlm.nih.gov/articles/PMC9676579/#) *and also* Fujiwara, Tomoko, et al., 'Skipping breakfast adversely affects menstrual disorders in young college students', *International Journal of Food Science and Nutrition,* 2009 (pubmed.ncbi.nlm.nih.gov/19468949/) *and also* Najafi, Nastaran, et al., 'Major dietary patterns in relation to menstrual pain: a nested case control study', *BMC Womens Health*, 21 May 2018 (pmc.ncbi.nlm.nih.gov/articles/PMC5963185/)

4. MoradiFili, Bahareh, et al., 'Dietary patterns are associated with premenstrual syndrome: evidence from a case-control study', *Public Health Nutrition*, 15 October 2019 (pubmed.ncbi.nlm.nih.gov/31612836/)
5. Rayanne E. Silva Noll, Priscilla, et al., 'Life habits of postmenopausal women: Association of menopause symptom intensity and food consumption by degree of food processing', *Maturitas*, February 2022 (pubmed.ncbi.nlm.nih.gov/35033227/#:~:)
6. Samuthpongtorn, Chatpol, MD, et al., 'Consumption of Ultraprocessed Food and Risk of Depression', *JAMA Network Open*, 20 September 2023 (https://jamanetwork.com/journals/jamanetworkopen/fullarticle/2809727)
7. Chang, Kiara, et al., 'Ultra-processed food consumption, cancer risk and cancer mortality: a large-scale prospective analysis within the UK Biobank', *The Lancet*, Volume 56, February 2023 (www.thelancet.com/journals/eclinm/article/PIIS2589-5370(23)00017-2/fulltext)
8. Walkyria, Paula O., et al., 'Maternal Consumption of Ultra-Processed Foods-Rich Diet and Perinatal Outcomes: A Systematic Review and Meta-Analysis', *Nutrients*, 8 August 2022 (pmc.ncbi.nlm.nih.gov/articles/PMC9370797/)
9. Henney, Alex E., et al., 'High intake of ultra-processed food is associated with dementia in adults: a systematic review and meta-analysis of observational studies', *Journal of Neurology*, January 2024 (pubmed.ncbi.nlm.nih.gov/37831127/)
10. Dunbar, R. I. M., 'Social eating connects communities', University of Oxford, 16 March 2017 (www.ox.ac.uk/news/2017-03-16-social-eating-connects-communities)
11. Future 50 Foods, Knorr and WWF, February 2019 (www.wwf.org.uk/sites/default/files/2019-02/Knorr_Future_50_Report_FINAL_Online.pdf)

ENDNOTES

Chapter 3. A woman's place

1. Boycott, Rosie, 'Why a woman's place is in the kitchen', *The Guardian*, 26 April 2007 (www.theguardian.com/world/2007/apr/26/gender.lifeandhealth)
2. Do Pico, Marina, 'Edward Bernays: The art of manipulation', *Digital Marketing*, 30 June 2023 (www.mdmarketingdigital.com/blog/en/edward-bernays-the-art-of-manipulation/)
3. Rudd Report, 'Targeted food and beverage advertising to Black and Hispanic consumers: 2022 update, November 2022 (uconnruddcenter.org/wp-content/uploads/sites/2909/2022/11/TargetedMarketing2022-Executive-Summary.pdf)
4. Kim, Dakota, 'A constant barrage: US companies target junk food ads to people of color', *The Guardian*, 11 November 2022 (www.theguardian.com/environment/2022/nov/11/junk-food-marketing-children-of-color)
5. O'Connor, Anahad, et al., 'The food industry pays "influencer" dietitians to shape your eating habits', *The Washington Post*, 13 September 2023 (www.washingtonpost.com/wellness/2023/09/13/dietitian-instagram-tiktok-paid-food-industry/)
6. Maguire, Lucy, et al., 'The *Vogue Business* AW24 size inclusivity report', *Vogue*, 11 March 2024 (www.voguebusiness.com/story/fashion/the-vogue-business-aw24-size-inclusivity-report)
7. Nanjo, Noor, 'Katie Price low-calorie diet advert for Skinny Food banned', BBC News, 3 April 2024 (www.bbc.co.uk/news/entertainment-arts-68713464)
8. Maynard, Maddie, 'Shopping habits: how do they differ between men and women?', *The Grocer*, 18 June 2021 (www.thegrocer.co.uk/analysis-and-features/shopping-habits-how-do-they-differ-between-men-and-women/656959.article)
9. Schaeffer, Katharine, 'Among U.S. couples, women do more cooking and grocery shopping than men', Pew Research Center, 24 September 2019 (www.pewresearch.

org/short-reads/2019/09/24/among-u-s-couples-women-do-more-cooking-and-grocery-shopping-than-men/)
10. Ibbetson, Connor, 'Do men do their fair share of housework?', YouGov, 7 February 2020 (yougov.co.uk/society/articles/27710-do-british-men-do-their-fair-share-housework)

Chapter 4. Start them young

1. Logan, Alan C., et al., '"Food faddists and pseudoscientists!": Reflections on the history of resistance to ultra-processed foods', *Explore*, Volume 20, Issue 4, July–August 2024 (www.sciencedirect.com/science/article/pii/S1550830723002847#bbib0082)
2. Freeland-Graves, Jeanne H., et al., 'Position of the Academy of Nutrition and Dietetics: Total Diet Approach to Healthy Eating', *Journal of the Academy of Nutrition and Dietetics*, Volume 113, Issue 2, February 2013 (www.jandonline.org/article/S2212-2672(12)01993-4/abstract)
3. Annual Report, 2015, Academy of Nutrition and Dietetics Foundation (https://web.archive.org/web/20160805162121/http://www.eatrightpro.org/~/media/eatrightpro%20files/about%20us/annual%20reports/annualreport2015.ashx#page=5)
4. Annual Report, 2021, Academy of Nutrition and Dietetics Foundation (www.eatrightpro.org/-/media/files/eatrightpro/about-us/annual-reports/2021_annual_report.pdf?)
5. Annual Report, 2022, Academy of Nutrition and Dietetics Foundation (www.eatrightpro.org/-/media/files/eatrightpro/about-us/annual-reports/2022-annual-report.pdf?)
6. Klemm, Sarah, 'Processed Foods: A Closer Look', Eat.right.org, 11 February 2019 (www.eatright.org/health/wellness/diet-trends/processed-foods-whats-ok-and-what-to-avoid)

ENDNOTES

7. 'Position statement on UPF, British Nutrition Foundation, 28 May 2024 (www.nutrition.org.uk/news/position-statement-on-the-concept-of-ultra-processed-foods-upf/)
8. Current Members, British Nutrition Foundation (www.nutrition.org.uk/who-we-work-with/current-members/), accessed September 2024, *and also* Chris van Tulleken, X, 27 April 2023 (x.com/DoctorChrisVT/status/1651525408733425664)
9. With thanks to Rob Percival at the Soil Association for this info. 'Sticky fingers of food industry on government ultra-processed food review', 11 July 2023 (www.soilassociation.org/blogs/2023/july/11/sticky-fingers-of-food-industry-on-government-ultra-processed-food-review/) *and also* 'UK government's nutrition advisers are paid by world's largest food companies', *BMJ*, 11 September 2024 (www.bmj.com/content/386/bmj.q1909)
10. Unicef, 'Blog: Supporting breastfeeding: we know what works; let's make it happen', 28 February 2017 (www.unicef.org.uk/babyfriendly/supporting-breastfeeding-make-it-happen/)
11. Sasson, Tehila, 'Milking the Third World? Humanitarianism, Capitalism, and the Moral Economy of the Nestlé Boycott', *The American Historical Review*, Volume 121, Issue 4, October 2016 (academic.oup.com/ahr/article/121/4/1196/2581604?) *and also* 'The Baby Killer', War on Want, March 1974 (waronwant.org/sites/default/files/THE%20BABY%20KILLER%201974.pdf)
12. Palmer, Gabrielle, *The Politics of Breastfeeding*, Pinter & Martin, 2011 *and also* 'The Baby Killer', War on Want, March 1974 (waronwant.org/sites/default/files/THE%20BABY%20KILLER%201974.pdf)
13. First Steps Nutrition Trust, 'Infant milks information for parents & carers' (www.firststepsnutrition.org/parents-carers), accessed September 2024

14. Taylor, Rosie, 'The toddler milks with more sugar than a chocolate milkshake – which are putting a THIRD of tots at risk of obesity and tooth decay', *Daily Mail*, 20 September 2024 (www.dailymail.co.uk/health/article-13875059/toddler-milks-sugar-chocolate-milkshake-obesity-tooth-decay.html)
15. Unicef, 'Breastfeeding in the UK' (www.unicef.org.uk/babyfriendly/about/breastfeeding-in-the-uk/), accessed September 2024
16. Aptamil, Breastfeeding (www.aptaclub.co.uk/feeding/breastfeeding.html), accessed September 2024
17. World Vision, 'Common Myths about Breastfeeding in Emergencies', 26 July 2023 (www.wvi.org/nutrition/article/common-myths-about-breastfeeding-emergencies)
18. Sisterhood of Motherhood (https://www.youtube.com/watch?v=Kz4BUwaxj5c)
19. Chu, Will, 'Infant nutrition: The business of "selling sleep" and "peace of mind"', NutraIngredients, 26 May 2017 (www.nutraingredients.com/Article/2017/05/16/Infant-nutrition-The-business-of-selling-sleep-and-peace-of-mind/) *and also* Rollins, Prof Nigel, et al., 'Marketing of commercial milk formula: a system to capture parents, communities, science, and policy', *The Lancet*, 11 February 2023 (www.sciencedirect.com/science/article/pii/S0140673622019316#bib59)
20. Rollins, Prof Nigel, et al., 'Marketing of commercial milk formula: a system to capture parents, communities, science, and policy', *The Lancet*, 11 February 2023 (www.thelancet.com/journals/lancet/article/PIIS0140-6736(22)01931-6/fulltext)
21. World Health Organization, 'Countries failing to stop harmful marketing of breast-milk substitutes, warn WHO and UNICEF', 27 May 2020 (www.who.int/news/item/27-05-2020-countries-failing-to-stop-harmful-marketing-of-breast-milk-substitutes-warn-who-and-unicef)

22. United Nations Sustainable Development Group, 'More African countries fight unethical marketing of breast-milk substitutes', 3 August 2022 (unsdg.un.org/latest/announcements/more-african-countries-fight-unethical-marketing-breast-milk-substitutes)
23. Newman, Melanie, and Wright, Oliver, 'After Nestlé, Aptamil manufacturer Danone is now hit by breast milk scandal', *The Independent*, 29 June 2013 (www.independent.co.uk/news/uk/home-news/after-nestle-aptamil-manufacturer-danone-is-now-hit-by-breast-milk-scandal-8679226.html)
24. Hausner, Helene, 'Breastfeeding facilitates acceptance of a novel dietary flavour compound', *Clinical Nutrition*, February 2010 (pubmed.ncbi.nlm.nih.gov/19962799/)
25. First Steps Nutrition, 'Ultra-Processed foods marketed for infants and young children in the UK' (www.firststepsnutrition.org/upfs-marketed-for-infants-and-young-children), accessed September 2024
26. University of Cambridge, 'Ultra-processed food makes up almost two-thirds of calorie intake of UK adolescents' (www.cam.ac.uk/research/news/ultra-processed-food-makes-up-almost-two-thirds-of-calorie-intake-of-uk-adolescents#), accessed September 2024
27. O'Hare, Ryan and Head, Emily, 'Ultra-processed foods make up almost two-thirds of Britain's school meals', Imperial, 30 July 2022 (www.imperial.ac.uk/news/238436/ultra-processed-foods-make-almost-two-thirds-britains/)
28. Obesity Action Coalition, 'Food marketing to Children: A Wolf in Sheep's Clothing?', Summer 2015 (www.obesityaction.org/resources/food-marketing-to-children-a-wolf-in-sheeps-clothing/)
29. Dos Santos Costa, Caroline, 'Consumption of ultra-processed foods and growth outcomes in early childhood: 2015 Pelotas Birth Cohort', *British Journal of Nutrition*, 28 June 2023 (pubmed.ncbi.nlm.nih.gov/36093936/)

30. World Health Organization, 'Noncommunicable diseases: Childhood overweight and obesity', 19 October 2020 (www.who.int/news-room/questions-and-answers/item/noncommunicable-diseases-childhood-overweight-and-obesity)
31. Khoury, Nadine, et al., 'Ultraprocessed Food Consumption and Cardiometabolic Risk Factors in Children', *Nutrition, Obesity, and Exercise*, 17 May 2024 (jamanetwork.com/journals/jamanetworkopen/fullarticle/2818951?)
32. Leffa, Paula, et al., 'Longitudinal associations between ultra-processed foods and blood lipids in childhood', *British Journal of Nutrition*, 14 August 2020 (pubmed.ncbi.nlm.nih.gov/32248849/)
33. Cascaes, Andreia Morales, et al., 'Ultra-processed food consumption and dental caries in children and adolescents: a systematic review and meta-analysis', *British Journal of Nutrition*, 27 July 2022 (pubmed.ncbi.nlm.nih.gov/35894293/)
34. Reales-Moreno, Marta, et al., 'Ultra-Processed Foods and Drinks Consumption Is Associated with Psychosocial Functioning in Adolescents', *Nutrients*, 15 November 2022 (pubmed.ncbi.nlm.nih.gov/36432518/)
35. Universitat Autònoma de Barcelona, 'Ultra-processed foods consumption with psychosocial problems associated with mental health in adolescents', 23 May 2023 (www.uab.cat/web/newsroom/news-detail/study-links-ultra-processed-foods-consumption-with-psychosocial-problems-associated-with-mental-health-in-adolescents-1345830290613.html)
36. Hayhoe, Richard, et al., 'Cross-sectional associations of schoolchildren's fruit and vegetable consumption, and meal choices, with their mental well-being: a cross-sectional study' *British Medical Journal*, 27 September 2021 (nutrition.bmj.com/content/early/2021/08/27/bmjnph-2020-000205)

37. Raine, Adrian and Brodrick, Lia, 'Omega-3 supplementation reduces aggressive behavior: A meta-analytic review of randomized controlled trials', *Science Direct*, September–October 2024 (www.sciencedirect.com/science/article/abs/pii/S13591789240004466)
38. World Health Organization, 'Just four industries cause 2.7 million deaths in the European Region every year', 12 June 2024 (www.who.int/europe/news/item/12-06-2024-just-four-industries-cause-2.7-million-deaths-in-the-european-region-every-year#:~)
39. Universitat Oberta de Catalunya, 'Eating in front of screens can lead to compulsive consumption of ultra-processed foods', 6 May 2024 (www.uoc.edu/en/news/2024/eating-in-front-of-screens-can-lead-to-compulsive-consumption-of-ultra-processed-foods)

Chapter 5. Ben? Jerry? I'm breaking up with you!

1. Campbell, Denis, 'More than half of humans on track to be overweight or obese by 2035', *The Guardian*, 2 March 2023 (www.theguardian.com/society/2023/mar/02/more-than-half-of-humans-on-track-to-be-overweight-or-obese-by-2035-report)
2. UK Parliament, Obesity Statistics, 12 January 2023 (commonslibrary.parliament.uk/research-briefings/sn03336/)
3. OECD, 'The future of health systems' (www.oecd.org/els/health-systems/Obesity-Update-2017.pdf), accessed September 2024
4. 'Worldwide trends in body-mass index, underweight, overweight, and obesity from 1975 to 2016: a pooled analysis of 2416 population-based measurement studies in 128·9 million children, adolescents, and adults', *The Lancet*, 16 December 2017 (www.thelancet.com/journals/lancet/article/PIIS0140-6736(17)32129-3/fulltext)

5. Kanter, Rebecca and Caballero, Benjamin, 'Global Gender Disparities in Obesity: A Review', *Advances in Nutrition*, Volume 3, Issue 4, July 2012 (www.sciencedirect.com/science/article/pii/S2161831322010249)
6. Humphrey, Jennifer L., 'Q & A with researcher Tera Fazzino: What to know about "hyperpalatable" foods', University of Kansas, 9 May 2023 (lifespan.ku.edu/q-researcher-tera-fazzino-what-know-about-hyperpalatable-foods)
7. Fazzino, Tera L., et al., 'US tobacco companies selectively disseminated hyper-palatable foods into the US food system: Empirical evidence and current implications', *Addiction*, Volume 119, Issue 1, 8 September 2023 (onlinelibrary.wiley.com/doi/10.1111/add.16332)
8. Fernandes, Ariana E., et al., 'Differences in the gut microbiota of women according to ultra-processed food consumption', *Nutrition, Metabolism and Cardiovascular Diseases*, January 2023 (pubmed.ncbi.nlm.nih.gov/36411218/)
9. Salame, Clara, et al., 'Food additive emulsifiers and the risk of type 2 diabetes: analysis of data from the NutriNet-Santé prospective cohort study', *The Lancet*, May 2024 (www.thelancet.com/journals/landia/article/PIIS2213-8587(24)00086-X/fulltext#:~)
10. Sellem, Laury, et al., 'Food additive emulsifiers and risk of cardiovascular disease in the NutriNet-Santé cohort: prospective cohort study', *British Medical Journal*, 6 September 2023 (www.bmj.com/content/382/bmj-2023-076058)
11. Cordova, Reynalda, et al., 'Consumption of ultra-processed foods and risk of multimorbidity of cancer and cardiometabolic diseases: a multinational cohort study', *The Lancet*, December 2023 (www.thelancet.com/journals/lanepe/article/PIIS2666-7762(23)00190-4/fulltext) ***and also*** Chang, Kiara, et al., 'Ultra-processed food consumption, cancer risk and cancer mortality: a large-scale prospective analysis within the UK Biobank', *The Lancet*, February

12. Özcan Dağ, Zeynep and Dilbaz, Berna, 'Impact of obesity on fertility in women', *Journal of the Turkish-German Gynecological Association*, 1 June 2015 (pmc.ncbi.nlm.nih.gov/articles/PMC4456969/)
13. Cancer Research UK, 'How does obesity cause cancer?' (www.cancerresearchuk.org/about-cancer/causes-of-cancer/bodyweight-and-cancer/how-does-obesity-cause-cancer), accessed September 2024
14. Breast Cancer Now, 'Weight, obesity and breast cancer' (breastcancernow.org/about-breast-cancer/awareness/breast-cancer-causes/weight-obesity-and-breast-cancer-risk/#), accessed September 2024
15. Chang, Kiara, et al. 'Ultra-processed food consumption, cancer risk and cancer mortality: a large-scale prospective analysis within the UK Biobank', *The Lancet*, February 2023 (www.thelancet.com/journals/eclinm/article/PIIS2589-5370(23)00017-2/fulltext)
16. Holdsworth-Carson, Sarah J., et al., 'The association of body mass index with endometriosis and disease severity in women with pain', *Journal of Endometriosis and Pelvic Pain Disorders*, 27 May 2018 (journals.sagepub.com/doi/abs/10.1177/2284026518773939)
17. Tang, Ruiyi, 'General and Central Obesity Are Associated With Increased Severity of the VMS and Sexual Symptoms of Menopause Among Chinese Women: A Longitudinal Study', *Endocrinology of Aging*, 26 April 2022 (www.frontiersin.org/journals/endocrinology/articles/10.3389/fendo.2022.814872/full#B9)
18. Lang, Katharine, 'Obesity may increase severity of menopause symptoms, make hormone therapy less effective', *Medical News Today*, 29 September 2023 (www.medicalnewstoday.com/articles/obesity-worsen-menopause-symptoms-reduce-hormone-therapy-efficacy)

19. Bailey, Eileen, 'Higher BMI is significantly associated with worse mental health, especially in women', *Medical News Today*, 6 March 2024 (www.medicalnewstoday.com/articles/higher-bmi-is-significantly-associated-with-worse-mental-health-especially-in-women#Results-from-the-high-BMI-and-mental-health-study) ***and also*** Simon, Gregory E., et al., 'Association between obesity and depression in middle-aged women', *General Hospital Psychiatry*, 30 April 2009 (www.ncbi.nlm.nih.gov/pmc/articles/PMC2675189/)
20. Li, Li, et al., 'Gender-Specific Relationship between Obesity and Major Depression', *Frontiers in Endocrinology*, 10 November 2017 (www.ncbi.nlm.nih.gov/pmc/articles/PMC5686049/)
21. Fernandes, Ariana E., et al., 'Differences in the gut microbiota of women according to ultra-processed food consumption', *Nutrition, Metabolism and Cardiovascular Disease*, January 2023 (pubmed.ncbi.nlm.nih.gov/36411218/)
22. Byth, Sophie, et al., 'The relationship between obesity and self-esteem: longitudinal evidence from Australian adults', *Oxford Open Economics*, 7 October 2022 (academic.oup.com/ooec/article/doi/10.1093/ooec/odac009/6751730)
23. Jun Ju, Yeong, et al., 'Association between weight control failure and suicidal ideation in overweight and obese adults: a cross-sectional study', *BMC Public Health*, 15 March 2016 (bmcpublichealth.biomedcentral.com/articles/10.1186/s12889-016-2940-1#:~)
24. Kolotkin, Ronette L., et al., 'Obesity and sexual quality of life', *Obesity*, March 2006 (pubmed.ncbi.nlm.nih.gov/16648619/)
25. *Ibid.*
26. Horstmann, Annette, et al., 'Obesity-Related Differences between Women and Men in Brain Structure and Goal-Directed Behavior', *Frontiers in Human Neuroscience*, June 2011 (www.researchgate.net/publication/51451934_Obesity-

Related_Differences_between_Women_and_Men_in_Brain_Structure_and_Goal-Directed_Behavior)

27. Udo, Tomoko, et al., 'Gender Differences in the Impact of Stressful Life Events on Changes in Body-Mass-Index', *Preventive Medicine*, 1 December 2015 (www.ncbi.nlm.nih.gov/pmc/articles/PMC4312235/) **and also** Guerrero-Hreins, Eva, et al., 'A Comparison of Emotional Triggers for Eating in Men and Women with Obesity', *Nutrients*, 6 October 2022 (www.ncbi.nlm.nih.gov/pmc/articles/PMC9570591/)

28. Gearhardt, Ashley N., et al., 'Social, clinical, and policy implications of ultra-processed food addiction', *British Medical Journal*, 9 October 2023 (www.bmj.com/content/383/bmj-2023-075354)

29. Thanarajah, Sharmili Edwin, et al., 'Habitual daily intake of a sweet and fatty snack modulates reward processing in humans', *Cell Metabolism*, 4 April 2023 (pubmed.ncbi.nlm.nih.gov/36958330/)

30. Figueiredo, Natasha, et al., 'Ultra-processed food intake and eating disorders: Cross-sectional associations among French adults', *Journal of Behavioral Addictions*, 4 April 2022 (www.ncbi.nlm.nih.gov/pmc/articles/PMC9295249/)

31. Ayton, Agnes, et al., 'Ultra-processed foods and binge eating: A retrospective observational study', *Nutrition*, April 2021 (www.sciencedirect.com/science/article/abs/pii/S0899900720303063)

32. Office for National Statistics, Child Abuse in England and Wales: March 2020 (www.ons.gov.uk/peoplepopulationandcommunity/crimeandjustice/bulletins/childabuseinenglandandwales/march2020#:~)

33. Caslini, Manuela, et al., 'Disentangling the Association Between Child Abuse and Eating Disorders: A Systematic Review and Meta-Analysis', *Psychosomatic Medicine*, January 2016 (pubmed.ncbi.nlm.nih.gov/26461853/) **and also** O'Loghlen, Elyse, et al., 'Childhood maltreatment, shame, psychological distress, and binge eating: testing a

serial mediational model', *Journal of Eating Disorders*, 13 June 2023 (jeatdisord.biomedcentral.com/articles/10.1186/s40337-023-00819-7)

34. Khazan, Olga, 'The Second Assault', *The Atlantic*, 15 December 2015 (www.theatlantic.com/health/archive/2015/12/sexual-abuse-victims-obesity/420186/)

35. Dugan, Nicholas, et al., 'Male gender is an independent risk factor for patients undergoing laparoscopic sleeve gastrectomy or Roux-en-Y gastric bypass: an MBSAQIP® database analysis', *Surgical Endoscopy*, 18 February 2020 (www.ncbi.nlm.nih.gov/pmc/articles/PMC7224103/#:~:text=Males%20continue%20to%20represent%20a,even%20after%20controlling%20for%20comorbidities)

36. Luthra, Shefali, 'Weight-loss drugs like Ozempic are more likely to interest women than men, poll finds', *The 19th*, 4 August 2023 (19thnews.org/2023/08/weight-loss-drugs-ozempic-women-poll/)

37. Helhoski, Anna, 'Will Ozempic Change the Food Industry? Not Yet, but Give It Time', *Nerdwallet*, 18 December 2023 (www.nerdwallet.com/article/finance/ozempic-glp1-food-industry)

38. British Nutrition, 'British Nutrition Foundation position statement on the concept of ultra-processed foods (UPF)', 28 May 2024 (www.nutrition.org.uk/news/position-statement-on-the-concept-of-ultra-processed-foods-upf/)

39. British Nutrition Foundation, Current Members (www.nutrition.org.uk/who-we-work-with/current-members/), accessed September 2024

40. Greenwood, George, 'Government "brainwashed" by fast-food lobbyists, ex-official says', *The Times*, 10 December 2023 (archive.ph/naflu#selection-2713.0-2715.115)

41. Greenwood, George, 'Revealed: KFC thwarting efforts to stop fast-food outlets near schools', *The Times*, 5 December 2023 (archive.ph/AcX3A)

ENDNOTES

42. Helmore, Edward, 'Lunchables with "improved nutrition" to be part of US school lunch programs', *The Guardian*, 14 March 2023 (www.theguardian.com/us-news/2023/mar/14/lunchables-school-lunch-programs)
43. Manley, Cameron, 'Kraft Heinz's CEO has a clean-eating lifestyle at odds with all that processed food – but he insists it shares his health mission', *Business Insider*, 27 April 2024 (www.businessinsider.com/kraft-heinz-ceo-health-habits-company-processed-products-2024-4)

Chapter 6. An apple a day keeps the OBGYN away

1. Mulak, Agata, et al., 'Sexual Dimorphism in the Gut Microbiome: Microgenderome or Microsexome?', *Journal of Neurogastroenterolgy and Motility*, 30 April 2022 (www.ncbi.nlm.nih.gov/pmc/articles/PMC8978118/)
2. Yuan, Xin, et al., 'Sexual dimorphism of gut microbiota at different pubertal status', *Microbial Cell Factories*, 28 July 2020 (pubmed.ncbi.nlm.nih.gov/32723385/)
3. Jašarević, Eldin, et al., 'Sex differences in the gut microbiome–brain axis across the lifespan', *Philosophical Transactions B*, 19 February 2016 (www.ncbi.nlm.nih.gov/pmc/articles/PMC4785905/)
4. Brennan, Caitriona, et al., 'Harnessing the power within: engineering the microbiome for enhanced gynecologic health', *Reproduction and Fertility*, 15 April 2024 (www.ncbi.nlm.nih.gov/pmc/articles/PMC11046331/)
5. Qin, Junjie, et al., 'A human gut microbial gene catalogue established by metagenomic sequencing', *Nature*, 4 March 2010 (pubmed.ncbi.nlm.nih.gov/20203603/)
6. Sonnenburg, Justin L. and Sonnenburg, Erica D., 'Vulnerability of the industrialized microbiota', *Science*, 25 October 2019 (www.science.org/doi/10.1126/science.aaw9255)

7. Miclotte, Lisa M.G., et al., 'Dietary emulsifiers alter composition and activity of the human gut microbiota in vitro, irrespective of chemical or natural emulsifier origin', ResearchGate, June 2020 (www.researchgate.net/publication/342526386_Dietary_emulsifiers_alter_composition_and_activity_of_the_human_gut_microbiota_in_vitro_irrespective_of_chemical_or_natural_emulsifier_origin)
8. Ruiz-Ojeda, Francisco Javier, et al., 'Effects of Sweeteners on the Gut Microbiota: A Review of Experimental Studies and Clinical Trials', *Advances in Nutrition*, January 2019 (www.sciencedirect.com/science/article/pii/S2161831322001983)
9. Zangara, Megan T., et al., 'Maltodextrin Consumption Impairs Intestinal Mucus Barrier and Accelerates Colitis Through Direct Actions on the Epithelium', *Frontiers in Immunology*, 14 March 2022 (www.frontiersin.org/journals/immunology/articles/10.3389/fimmu.2022.841188/full)
10. Ostrowski, Matthew P., et al., 'Mechanistic insights into consumption of the food additive xanthan gum by the human gut microbiota', *Nature Microbiology*, April 2022 (pubmed.ncbi.nlm.nih.gov/35365790/)
11. Whelan, Kevin, et al., 'Ultra-processed foods and food additives in gut health and disease', *Nature Reviews*, 22 February 2024 (www.nature.com/articles/s41575-024-00893-5)
12. Elkafas, Hoda, et al., 'Gut and genital tract microbiomes: Dysbiosis and link to gynecological disorders', *Frontiers in Cellular and Infection Microbiology*, 16 December 2022 (www.ncbi.nlm.nih.gov/pmc/articles/PMC9800796/#B81)
13. Kwang Ng, Beng, et al., 'Maternal and fetal outcomes of pregnant women with bacterial vaginosis', *Frontiers*, 13 February 2023 (www.frontiersin.org/articles/10.3389/fsurg.2023.1084867/full#:~)
14. Noormohammadi, Morvarid, et al., 'Association between dietary patterns and bacterial vaginosis: a case–control study',

Scientific Reports, 16 July 2022 (www.ncbi.nlm.nih.gov/pmc/articles/PMC9288476/)

15. Brennan, Caitriona, et al., 'Harnessing the Power Within: Engineering the Microbiome for Enhanced Gynecologic Health', March 2024 (www.researchgate.net/publication/379062428_Harnessing_the_Power_Within_Engineering_the_Microbiome_for_Enhanced_Gynecologic_Health)

16. Stapleton, Ann E., 'The Vaginal Microbiota and Urinary Tract Infection', *Microbiology Spectrum Journal*, 29 December 2017 (https://pmc.ncbi.nlm.nih.gov/articles/PMC5746606/#:~)

17. Barnard, Neal D., et al., 'Nutrition in the prevention and treatment of endometriosis: A review', *Frontiers in Nutrition*, 17 February 2023 (www.ncbi.nlm.nih.gov/pmc/articles/PMC9983692/#:~)

18. Rossler, Hannah, et al., 'Alterations of the gut microbiota in borderline personality disorder', *Journal of Psychosomatic Research*, 13 May 2022 (pubmed.ncbi.nlm.nih.gov/35594813/)

19. Maeng, Lisa Y., and Beumer, Amy, 'Never fear, the gut bacteria are here: Estrogen and gut microbiome-brain axis interactions in fear extinction', *International Journal of Psychophysiology*, July 2023 (www.sciencedirect.com/science/article/pii/S0167876023004300#)

20. Yao, Yao, et al., 'The Role of Microbiota in Infant Health: From Early Life to Adulthood', *Frontiers in Immunology*, 7 October 2021 (www.frontiersin.org/journals/immunology/articles/10.3389/fimmu.2021.708472/full#B57)

21. Toson, Bruno, et al., 'The Endometrial Microbiome and its Impact on Human Conception', *International Journal of Molecular Science*, 1 January 2022 (www.ncbi.nlm.nih.gov/pmc/articles/PMC8745284/#:~)

22. Chanomethaporn, Anchana, et al., 'Association between periodontitis and spontaneous abortion: A case-control

study', *Journal of Periodontology*, April 2019 (pubmed.ncbi. nlm.nih.gov/30367824/)

23. Daalderop, L. A., et al., 'Periodontal Disease and Pregnancy Outcomes: Overview of Systematic Reviews', *JDR Clinical & Translational Research*, January 2018 (pubmed.ncbi.nlm.nih. gov/30370334/)

24. Zhu Jun, et al., 'The association of gut microbiome with recurrent pregnancy loss: A comprehensive review', *Drug Discoveries & Therapeutics*, June 2025 (pubmed.ncbi.nlm. nih.gov/37357394/)

25. Sonnenburg, Justin and Gardner, Christopher, 'Fermented Foods, Fibre, and Immunity', Episode 191 (theproof. com/fermented-foods-fibre-and-immunity-with-dr-justin-sonnenburg-dr-christopher-gardner/)

26. National Institute of Environmental Health Sciences, 'Inflammation' (www.niehs.nih.gov/health/topics/conditions/ inflammation#:~), accessed September 2024

27. Stanford Medicine, 'Gut-Microbiota-Targeted Diets Modulate Human Immune Status: Fe-Fi-Fo Study', August 2021 (med. stanford.edu/nutrition/research/completed-studies/fefifo.html)

28. Zidan, Souzan, et al., 'Could psychobiotics and fermented foods improve mood in middle-aged and older women?' *Maturitas*, March 2024 (www.sciencedirect.com/science/ article/abs/pii/S0378512223005091)

29. Tillisch, Kirsten, et al. 'Consumption of fermented milk product with probiotic modulates brain activity', *Gastroenterology*, June 2013 (pubmed.ncbi.nlm.nih. gov/23474283/)

30. Suez, Jotham, et al., 'Post-Antibiotic Gut Mucosal Microbiome Reconstitution Is Impaired by Probiotics and Improved by Autologous FMT', 6 September 2018 (pubmed. ncbi.nlm.nih.gov/30193113/) ***and also*** Wastyk, Hannah C., et al., 'Randomized controlled trial demonstrates response to a probiotic intervention for metabolic syndrome that may correspond to diet', *Gut Microbes*, 28 July 2022

(www.tandfonline.com/doi/full/10.1080/19490976.2023.2178794) *and also* (www.evidentlycochrane.net/probiotics-prebiotics-synbiotics-the-evidence-behind-the-claims/#:~)

Chapter 7. Unlucky women?

1. Hardwicke Collings, Jane, 'Introducing Sagescence' (janehardwickecollings.com/introducing-sagescence/), accessed September 2024
2. Gamble, Jessa, 'Early Starters', *Nature*, 5 October 2017 (www.nature.com/articles/550S10a)
3. Rees, M., 'The age of menarche', 1995 (pubmed.ncbi.nlm.nih.gov/12319855/)
4. Sole-Smith, Virginia, 'Why Are Girls Getting Their Periods So Young', *Scientific American*, 1 May 2019 (www.scientificamerican.com/article/why-are-girls-getting-their-periods-so-young/)
5. Moorhead, Joanna, 'Should we be worried about early puberty?', *The Guardian*, 19 October 2010 (www.theguardian.com/lifeandstyle/2010/oct/19/worried-about-early-puberty)
6. Weir, Kirsten, 'The risks of earlier puberty', American Psychological Association, March 2016 (www.apa.org/monitor/2016/03/puberty)
7. 'Menarche, menopause, and breast cancer risk: individual participant meta-analysis, including 118 964 women with breast cancer from 117 epidemiological studies', *The Lancet*, November 2012 (pubmed.ncbi.nlm.nih.gov/23084519/)
8. Soliman, Ashraf, et al., 'Nutrition and pubertal development', *Indian Journal of Endocrinology and Metabolism*, November 2014 (www.ncbi.nlm.nih.gov/pmc/articles/PMC4266867/#:~)
9. Harvard School of Public Health, 'Sugary drinks linked with earlier menstruation' (www.hsph.harvard.edu/news/hsph-in-the-news/sugary-drinks-linked-with-earlier-menstruation/) *and also* Carwile, J. L., 'Sugar-sweetened beverage

consumption and age at menarche in a prospective study of US girls', *Human Reproduction*, March 2015 (pubmed.ncbi.nlm.nih.gov/25628346/)

10. Tsai, Meng-Che, et al., 'Association of the consumption of common drinks with early puberty in both sexes', *Frontiers in Public Health*, 2 December 2022 (www.ncbi.nlm.nih.gov/pmc/articles/PMC9758723/)

11. Duan, Ruonan, et al., 'Modern dietary pattern is prospectively associated with earlier age at menarche: data from the CHNS 1997–2015', *Nutrition Journal*, 9 September 2020 (www.ncbi.nlm.nih.gov/pmc/articles/PMC7488069/)

12. Szamreta, Elizabeth A., et al., 'Greater adherence to a Mediterranean-like diet is associated with later breast development and menarche in peripubertal girls', *Public Health Nutrition*, 23 August 2019 (pmc.ncbi.nlm.nih.gov/articles/PMC10071494/#:~)

13. Endometriosis UK, 'It takes an average 7.5 years to get a diagnosis of endometriosis – it shouldn't' (www.endometriosis-uk.org/it-takes-average-75-years-get-diagnosis-endometriosis-it-shouldnt), accessed September 2024

14. NHS, 'Heavy periods' (www.nhs.uk/conditions/heavy-periods/)

15. The Conversation, 'Ultra-processed foods: it's not just their low nutritional value that's a concern', 12 September 2022 (theconversation.com/ultra-processed-foods-its-not-just-their-low-nutritional-value-thats-a-concern-189918)

16. Myles, Ian A., 'Fast food fever: reviewing the impacts of the Western diet on immunity', *Nutrition Journal*, 17 June 2014 (pubmed.ncbi.nlm.nih.gov/24939238/)

17. Onieva-Zafra, Maria Dolores, et al., 'Relationship Between Diet, Menstrual Pain and Other Menstrual Characteristics among Spanish Students', *Nutrients*, 2020 (www.mdpi.com/2072-6643/12/6/1759)

ENDNOTES

18. Najafi, Nastaran, et al., 'Major dietary patterns in relation to menstrual pain: a nested case control study', *BMC Womens Health*, 21 May 2018 (www.ncbi.nlm.nih.gov/pmc/articles/PMC5963185/#CR27) **and also** Fujiwara, Tomoko, et al., 'Skipping breakfast adversely affects menstrual disorders in young college students', *International Journal of Food Sciences and Nutrition*, 2009 (www.tandfonline.com/doi/full/10.1080/09637480802260998)
19. Hashim, Mona S., et al., 'Premenstrual Syndrome is Associated with Dietary and Lifestyle Behaviors Among University Students: A Cross-Sectional Study from Sharjah, UAE', *Nutrients*, 17 August 2019 (pubmed.ncbi.nlm.nih.gov/31426498/)
20. MoradiFili, Bahareh, et al., 'Dietary patterns are associated with premenstrual syndrome: evidence from a case-control study', *Public Health Nutrition*, April 2020 (pubmed.ncbi.nlm.nih.gov/31612836/)
21. Shoaibinobarian, Nargeskhatoon, et al., 'Association between ultra-processed foods and polycystic ovary syndrome: a case-control study', ResearchGate, January 2022 (www.researchgate.net/publication/364224910_Association_between_ultra-processed_foods_and_polycystic_ovary_syndrome_a_case-control_study)
22. Valle-Hita, Cristina, et al., 'Ultra-processed food consumption and semen quality parameters in the Led-Fertyl study', *Human Reproduction Open*, 17 January 2024 (pubmed.ncbi.nlm.nih.gov/38283622/#:~)
23. Lv, Jia-Le, et al., 'Intake of ultra-processed foods and asthenozoospermia odds: A hospital-based case-control study', *Frontiers in Nutrition*, 20 October 2022 (www.ncbi.nlm.nih.gov/pmc/articles/PMC9630735/)
24. Afeiche, Myriam C., et al., 'Processed Meat Intake is Unfavorably and Fish Intake Favorably Associated with Semen Quality Indicators among Men Attending a Fertility Clinic', *The Journal of Nutrition*, 21 May 2014 (www.ncbi.

nlm.nih.gov/pmc/articles/PMC4056648/) ***and also*** Xia, Wei, et al., 'Men's meat intake and treatment outcomes among couples undergoing assisted reproduction', *Fertility and Sterility*, October 2015 (pubmed.ncbi.nlm.nih.gov/26206344/)

25. Chavarro, Jorge E., et al., 'Soy food and isoflavone intake in relation to semen quality parameters among men from an infertility clinic', *Human Reproduction*, 23 July 2008 (www.ncbi.nlm.nih.gov/pmc/articles/PMC2721724/)

26. Whittaker, Joseph, 'Dietary trends and the decline in male reproductive health', *Hormones*, June 2023 (pubmed.ncbi.nlm.nih.gov/36725796/)

27. Skoracka, Kinga, et al., 'Diet and Nutritional Factors in Male (In)fertility – Underestimated Factors', *Journal of Clinical Medicine*, 9 May 2020 (www.ncbi.nlm.nih.gov/pmc/articles/PMC7291266/)

28. BBC, 'How pollution is causing a male fertility crisis', 28 March 2023 (www.bbc.com/future/article/20230327-how-pollution-is-causing-a-male-fertility-crisis)

29. Zhang, Chenming, et al., 'Microplastics May Be a Significant Cause of Male Infertility', *American Journal of Men's Health*, 24 May 2022 (www.ncbi.nlm.nih.gov/pmc/articles/PMC9134445/)

30. Hande Çekici, Hande, and Akdevelioğlu, Yasemin, 'The association between trans fatty acids, infertility and fetal life: a review', *Human Fertility*, 4 November 2017 (www.tandfonline.com/doi/full/10.1080/14647273.2018.1432078)

31. Skoracka, Kinga, et al., 'Female Fertility and the Nutritional Approach: The Most Essential Aspects', *Advances in Nutrition*, November 2021 (www.sciencedirect.com/science/article/pii/S2161831322005129?)

32. Rauber, Fernanda, et al., 'Ultra-processed food consumption and indicators of obesity in the United Kingdom population (2008-2016)', 1 May 2020 (journals.plos.org/plosone/article?id=10.1371/journal.pone.0232676)

33. Grieger, Jessica, et al., 'Pre-pregnancy fast food and fruit intake is associated with time to pregnancy', *Human Reproduction*, June 2018 (academic.oup.com/humrep/article/33/6/1063/4989162)
34. Kudesia, Rashmi, et al., 'Dietary Approaches to Women's Sexual and Reproductive Health', *American Journal of Lifestyle Medicine*, 8 May 2021 (www.ncbi.nlm.nih.gov/pmc/articles/PMC8299929/#bibr33-15598276211007113)
35. Lorenz, Tierney A., 'Interactions between inflammation and female sexual desire and arousal function', *Current Sex Health Reports*, 11 December 2011 (www.ncbi.nlm.nih.gov/pmc/articles/PMC7731354/)
36. Cai, Tommaso, et al., 'Apple consumption is related to better sexual quality of life in young women', *Archives of Gynecology and Obstetrics*, 12 February 2014 (pubmed.ncbi.nlm.nih.gov/24518938/)
37. University of Oxford, 'Autoimmune disorders found to affect around one in ten people' (www.ox.ac.uk/news/2023-05-06-autoimmune-disorders-found-affect-around-one-ten-people), accessed September 2024
38. Klein, Sabra L., and Flanagan, Katie L., 'Sex differences in immune responses', *Nature Reviews Immunology*, 22 August 2016 (www.nature.com/articles/nri.2016.90)
39. The Francis Crick Institute, 'World Immunology Day: Autoimmunity: when your immune system turns on you' (www.crick.ac.uk/whats-on/world-immunology-day-autoimmunity-when-your-immune-system-turns-on-you), accessed September 2024
40. Stanford Medicine, 'Stanford Medicine-led study shows why women are at greater risk of autoimmune disease', 1 February 2024 (med.stanford.edu/news/all-news/2024/02/women-autoimmune.html)
41. McKie, Robin, 'Global spread of autoimmune disease blamed on western diet', *The Guardian*, 9 January 2022 (www.

theguardian.com/science/2022/jan/08/global-spread-of-autoimmune-disease-blamed-on-western-diet)

42. Rossato, Sinara, et al., 'Ultraprocessed Food Intake and Risk of Systemic Lupus Erythematosus Among Women Observed in the Nurses' Health Study Cohorts', *Arthritis Care and Research*, 27 June 2024 (pubmed.ncbi.nlm.nih.gov/38937143/)

43. Narula, Neeraj, et al., 'Association of ultra-processed food intake with risk of inflammatory bowel disease: prospective cohort study', *BMJ*, 15 July 2021 (www.bmj.com/content/374/bmj.n1554) *and also* Lo, Chun-Han, et al., 'Ultra-processed Foods and Risk of Crohn's Disease and Ulcerative Colitis: A Prospective Cohort Study',*Clinical Gastroenterology and Hepatology*, June 2022 (pubmed.ncbi.nlm.nih.gov/34461300)
and also Narula, Neeraj, et al., 'Food Processing and Risk of Inflammatory Bowel Disease: A Systematic Review and Meta-Analysis', *Clinical Gastroenterology and Hepatology*, September 2023 (www.sciencedirect.com/science/article/abs/pii/S154235652300071X#:~)

44. Silva, Ana Rita, et al., 'An anti-inflammatory and low fermentable oligo, di, and monosaccharides and polyols diet improved patient reported outcomes in fibromyalgia: A randomized controlled trial', *Frontiers in Nutrition*, 15 August 2022 (www.ncbi.nlm.nih.gov/pmc/articles/PMC9450131/)

45. Smith, Jerry D., et al., 'Relief of Fibromyalgia Symptoms following Discontinuation of Dietary Excitotoxins', *Annals of Pharmacotherapy*, June 2001 (journals.sagepub.com/doi/10.1345/aph.10254)

46. Mazzucca, Camilla Barbero, et al., 'Nutrition and Rheumatoid Arthritis Onset: A Prospective Analysis Using the UK Biobank', *Nutrients*, 8 April 2022 (www.ncbi.nlm.nih.gov/pmc/articles/PMC9025922/)

47. Smaira, Fabiana Infante, et al., 'Ultra-processed food consumption associates with higher cardiovascular risk in rheumatoid arthritis', *Clinical Rheumatology*, May 2020 (pubmed.ncbi.nlm.nih.gov/31902026/)
48. Guglielmetti, Monica, et al., 'Ultra-processed foods consumption is associated with multiple sclerosis severity', *Frontiers in Neurology*, 24 January 2023 (www.ncbi.nlm.nih.gov/pmc/articles/PMC9902937/)
49. De Luca, F., and Shoenfeld, Y., 'The microbiome in autoimmune diseases', *Clinical & Experimental Immunology*, 19 December 2018 (www.ncbi.nlm.nih.gov/pmc/articles/PMC6300652/) *and also* Szamreta, Elizabeth A., et al., 'Greater adherence to a Mediterranean-like diet is associated with later breast development and menarche in peripubertal girls', *Public Health Nutrition*, 23 August 2019 (pmc.ncbi.nlm.nih.gov/articles/PMC10071494/#:~)
50. Today's Dietitian, 'Possible Link Between Processed Foods and Autoimmune Diseases', (www.todaysdietitian.com/news/031816_news.shtml) *and also* '"Likely Culprit" in Celiac Disease Hidden in Processed Foods', *Medium* (truthinlabeling.medium.com/likely-culprit-in-celiac-disease-hidden-in-processed-foods-4650232a8f21) *and also* Lerner, Aaron, et al., 'Cross-reactivity and sequence similarity between microbial transglutaminase and human tissue antigens', *Scientific Reports*, 16 October 2023 (www.ncbi.nlm.nih.gov/pmc/articles/PMC10579360/, accessed September 2024
51. Templeton, A., 'Obesity and Women's Health', *Facts, Views and Vision*, 2014 (pmc.ncbi.nlm.nih.gov/articles/PMC4286855/)
52. Paula, Walkyria, et al., 'Maternal Consumption of Ultra-Processed Foods-Rich Diet and Perinatal Outcomes: A Systematic Review and Meta-Analysis', *Nutrients*, 8 August 2022 (www.ncbi.nlm.nih.gov/pmc/articles/PMC9370797/)

53. University of Birmingham, 'Diet high in fruit and vegetables linked to lower miscarriage risk', 19 April 2023 (www.birmingham.ac.uk/news/2023/diet-high-in-fruit-and-vegetables-linked-to-lower-miscarriage-risk#:~)
54. Smit, Ashley J. P., et al., 'A high periconceptional maternal ultra-processed food consumption impairs embryonic growth: The Rotterdam periconceptional cohort', *Clinical Nutrition*, August 2022 (www.clinicalnutritionjournal.com/article/S0261-5614(22)00189-3/fulltext)
55. Hatzlhoffer Lourenço, Bárbara, et al., 'Exposure to ultra-processed foods during pregnancy and ultrasound fetal growth parameters', *British Journal of Nutrition*, 16 May 2023 (pubmed.ncbi.nlm.nih.gov/37190988/)
56. Swan, S. H., et al., 'First trimester phthalate exposure and anogenital distance in newborns', *Human Reproduction*, April 2015 (academic.oup.com/humrep/article/30/4/963/613595)
57. Ben-Avraham, Sivan, et al., 'Ultra-processed food (UPF) intake in pregnancy and maternal and neonatal outcomes', *European Journal of Nutrition*, 6 January 2023 (link.springer.com/article/10.1007/s00394-022-03072-x)
58. Baker, Brennan H., et al., 'Ultra-processed and fast food consumption, exposure to phthalates during pregnancy, and socioeconomic disparities in phthalate exposures', *Environment International*, January 2024 (www.sciencedirect.com/science/article/pii/S0160412024000138)
59. Halldorsson, Thorhallur, et al., 'Intake of artificially sweetened soft drinks and risk of preterm delivery: a prospective cohort study in 59,334 Danish pregnant women', *American Journal of Clinical Nutrition*, September 2010 (pubmed.ncbi.nlm.nih.gov/20592133/)
60. Englund-Ögge, Linda, et al., 'Association between intake of artificially sweetened and sugar-sweetened beverages and preterm delivery: a large prospective cohort study', *American*

Journal of Clinical Nutrition, September 2012 (pubmed.ncbi. nlm.nih.gov/22854404/)

61. Tollånes, Mette C., et al., 'Intake of Caffeinated Soft Drinks Before and During Pregnancy, but Not Total Caffeine Intake, is Associated with Increased Cerebral Palsy Risk in the Norwegian Mother and Child Cohort Study', *Journal of Nutrition*, September 2016 (pubmed.ncbi.nlm.nih. gov/27489007/)

62. Wright, Lakiea S., et al., 'Prenatal and Early Life Fructose, Fructose-Containing Beverages, and Midchildhood Asthma', *Annals of the American Thoracic Society*, 8 December 2017 (www.atsjournals.org/doi/full/10.1513/AnnalsATS.201707-530OC) **and also** Hamdan Al-Zalabani, Abdulmohsen, et al., 'Association between soft drinks consumption and asthma: a systematic review and meta-analysis', *BMJ Open*, 14 October 2019 (pubmed.ncbi.nlm.nih.gov/31615794/)

63. Grønning Dale, Maria, et al., 'Intake of sucrose-sweetened soft beverages during pregnancy and risk of congenital heart defects (CHD) in offspring: a Norwegian pregnancy cohort study', *European Journal of Epidemiology*, April 2019 (pubmed.ncbi.nlm.nih.gov/30661159/)

64. Rodríguez-Cano, Ameyalli, et al., 'Ultra-Processed Food Consumption during Pregnancy and Its Association with Maternal Oxidative Stress Markers', *Antioxidants*, 21 July 2022 (www.ncbi.nlm.nih.gov/pmc/articles/PMC9312096/)

65. Duhig, Kate, et al., 'Oxidative stress in pregnancy and reproduction', *Obstetric Medicine*, 17 May 2016 (www.ncbi. nlm.nih.gov/pmc/articles/PMC5010123/)

66. Puig-Vallverdú, Julia, et al., 'The association between maternal ultra-processed food consumption during pregnancy and child neuropsychological development: A population-based birth cohort study', *Clinical Nutrition*, October 2022 (pubmed.ncbi.nlm.nih.gov/36087519/)

67. Wang, Yiqing, 'Maternal consumption of ultra-processed foods and subsequent risk of offspring overweight or obesity:

results from three prospective cohort studies', *BMJ*, 5 October 2022 (www.bmj.com/content/379/bmj-2022-071767#:~)

Chapter 8. I'll have the blues

1. Food and Mood Centre (foodandmoodcentre.com.au/), accessed September 2024
2. Tasca, Cecilia, et al. 'Women and Hysteria in the History of Mental Health', *Clinical Practice and Epidemiology in Mental Health*, 19 October 2012 (www.ncbi.nlm.nih.gov/pmc/articles/PMC3480686/#:~)
3. Future Care Capital, 'Young women who ask for mental health help are called "dramatic", survey finds', 17 July 2023 (futurecarecapital.org.uk/latest/womens-mental-health-not-taken-seriously/)
4. Campaign Against Living Miserably, 'The signs women are struggling are going unseen. Meet the people fighting for change', 16 July 2023 (www.thecalmzone.net/unseen-signals/meet-the-people-fighting-for-change)
5. Albert, Paul A., 'Why is depression more prevalent in women?', *Journal of Psychiatry & Neuroscience*, July 2015 (www.ncbi.nlm.nih.gov/pmc/articles/PMC4478054/)
6. *Ibid.*
7. Witters, Dan, 'US Depression Rates Reach New highs', Gallup, 17 May 2023 (news.gallup.com/poll/505745/depression-rates-reach-new-highs.aspx#:~)
8. Cooney, Julene Kemp, 'Suicide Rates Have Soared Among Middle-Aged White Women in the US', Syracuse University, March 2019 (www.maxwell.syr.edu/research/lerner-center/population-health-research-brief-series/article/suicide-rates-have-soared-among-middle-aged-white-women-in-the-us)
9. Census 2021, 'Suicides in England and Wales: 2021 registrations' (www.ons.gov.uk/peoplepopulationandcommunity/birthsdeathsandmarriages/deaths/bulletins/suicidesintheunitedkingdom/2021registrations)

ENDNOTES

10. Campaign Against Living Miserably, 'The signs women are struggling are going unseen. Meet the people fighting for change', 16 July 2023 (www.thecalmzone.net/unseen-signals/meet-the-people-fighting-for-change)
11. Samuthpongtorn, Chatpol, et al., 'Consumption of Ultraprocessed Food and Risk of Depression', JAMA, 20 September 2023 (jamanetwork.com/journals/jamanetworkopen/fullarticle/2809727)
12. LaMotte, Sandee, 'Artificially sweetened ultraprocessed foods linked to depression in women, study finds', *CNN Health*, 20 September 2023 (edition.cnn.com/2023/09/20/health/no-calorie-ultraprocessed-food-depression-wellness/index.html)
13. Dai, Shuhui, et al., 'Ultra-processed foods and human health: An umbrella review and updated meta-analyses of observational evidence', *Clinical Nutrition*, June 2024 (www.sciencedirect.com/science/article/pii/S0261561424001225)
14. Jones, Sara K., et al., 'Transgenerational transmission of aspartame-induced anxiety and changes in glutamate-GABA signaling and gene expression in the amygdala', *Neuroscience*, 27 October 2022 (www.pnas.org/doi/10.1073/pnas.2213120119)
15. Meller, Fernanda Oliveira, et al., 'Consumption of ultra-processed foods and mental health of pregnant women from the South of Brazil', *British Journal of Nutrition*, 14 July 2024 (pubmed.ncbi.nlm.nih.gov/38644622/)
16. The Conversation, 'For women with antenatal depression, micronutrients might help them and their babies – new study', 3 June 2024 (theconversation.com/for-women-with-antenatal-depression-micronutrients-might-help-them-and-their-babies-new-study-228097)
17. Collet, Ophélie A., et al., 'Prenatal Diet and Children's Trajectories of Anxiety and Depression Symptoms from 3 to 8 Years: The EDEN Mother-Child Cohort', *Journal*

of Nutrition, 4 January 2021 (pubmed.ncbi.nlm.nih.gov/33296456/#:~)

18. Oddo, Vanessa M., et al., 'Mediterranean Diet Adherence and Depressive Symptoms among a Nationally Representative Sample of Pregnant Women in the United States', *The Journal of Nutrition*, October 2023 (www.sciencedirect.com/science/article/abs/pii/S0022316623725509?via%3Dihub)

19. Chatzi, Leda, et al., 'Dietary patterns during pregnancy and the risk of postpartum depression: the mother–child 'Rhea' cohort in Crete, Greece', Cambridge University Press, 11 April 2011 (www.cambridge.org/core/journals/public-health-nutrition/article/dietary-patterns-during-pregnancy-and-the-risk-of-postpartum-depression-the-motherchild-rhea-cohort-in-crete-greece/423D42D06D7F75199A307300E765EFC8)

20. Dehghan-Banadaki, Shima, et al., 'Empirically derived dietary patterns and postpartum depression symptoms in a large sample of Iranian women', *BMC Psychiatry*, June 2023 (www.ncbi.nlm.nih.gov/pmc/articles/PMC10261841/#:~)

21. Lane, Melissa M., et al., 'Ultra-processed food exposure and adverse health outcomes: umbrella review of epidemiological meta-analyses', *BMJ*, 28 February 2024 (www.bmj.com/content/384/bmj-2023-077310)

22. Lane, Melissa M., et al., 'Ultra-processed food exposure and adverse health outcomes: umbrella review of epidemiological meta-analyses', *BMJ*, 28 February 2024 (www.bmj.com/content/384/bmj-2023-077310) **and also** US Right to Know, 'Ultra-processed foods: increased risk of depression and anxiety' (usrtk.org/ultra-processed-foods/depression-anxiety/#:~) **and also** Ejtahed, Hanieh-Sadat, et al., 'Association between junk food consumption and mental health problems in adults: a systematic review and meta-analysis', *BMC Psychiatry*, 12 June 2024 (bmcpsychiatry.biomedcentral.com/articles/10.1186/s12888-024-05889-8#:~)

23. Sapien Labs, 'Consumption of ultra-processed food and wellbeing outcomes', 2 October 2023 (sapienlabs.org/

consumption-of-ultra-processed-food-and-mental-wellbeing-outcomes/)
24. Werneck, André O., et al., 'Adherence to the ultra-processed dietary pattern and risk of depressive outcomes: Findings from the NutriNet Brasil cohort study and an updated systematic review and meta-analysis', *Clinical Nutrition*, May 2024 (www.clinicalnutritionjournal.com/article/S0261-5614(24)00102-X/abstract)
25. Adjibade, Moufidath, et al., 'Prospective association between ultra-processed food consumption and incident depressive symptoms in the French NutriNet-Santé cohort', *BMC Medicine*, 15 April 2019 (bmcmedicine.biomedcentral.com/articles/10.1186/s12916-019-1312-y)
26. Food and Mood Centre (foodandmoodcentre.com.au/smiles-trial/) *and also* Jacka, Felice N., et al., 'A randomised controlled trial of dietary improvement for adults with major depression (the "SMILES" trial)', *BMC Medicine*, 30 January 2017 (www.ncbi.nlm.nih.gov/pmc/articles/PMC5282719/)
27. Nanri, Akiko, et al., 'Dietary patterns and suicide in Japanese adults: the Japan Public Health Center-based Prospective Study', *British Journal of Psychiatry*, December 2013 (pubmed.ncbi.nlm.nih.gov/24115342/)
28. Mansuy-Aubert, Virginie and Ravussin, Yann, 'Short chain fatty acids: the messengers from down below', *Frontiers of Neuroscience*, 6 July 2021 (www.frontiersin.org/journals/neuroscience/articles/10.3389/fnins.2023.1197759/full)
29. O'Neil, Adrienne, et al., 'The association between poor dental health and depression: findings from a large-scale, population-based study (the NHANES study)', *General Hospital Psychiatry*, May–June 2014 (www.sciencedirect.com/science/article/abs/pii/S0163834314000139)
30. Wingfield, Benjamin, et al., 'Variations in the oral microbiome are associated with depression in young adults', *Nature*, 22 July 2021 (www.nature.com/articles/s41598-021-94498-6) *and also* Li, Chun'e, et al., 'A genetic association study

reveals the relationship between the oral microbiome and anxiety and depression symptoms', *Behavioral and Psychiatric Genetics*, 10 November 2022 (www.frontiersin.org/journals/psychiatry/articles/10.3389/fpsyt.2022.960756/full#B1)

31. Xiong, Ruo-Gu, et al., 'The Role of Gut Microbiota in Anxiety, Depression, and Other Mental Disorders as Well as the Protective Effects of Dietary Components', *Nutrients*, 23 July 2023 (www.ncbi.nlm.nih.gov/pmc/articles/PMC10384867/)

32. Niemela, Leila, et al., 'Exploring gender differences in the relationship between gut microbiome and depression – a scoping review', *Frontiers of Psychiatry*, 19 February 2024 (www.frontiersin.org/journals/psychiatry/articles/10.3389/fpsyt.2024.1361145/full)

33. Cuevas-Sierra, Amanda, et al., 'Gut Microbiota Differences According to Ultra-Processed Food Consumption in a Spanish Population', *Nutrients*, 2021 (www.mdpi.com/2072-6643/13/8/2710#)

34. Dinan, Timothy G., 'How do gut microbes influence mental health?', *Microbiome*, 16 May 2022 (wchh.onlinelibrary.wiley.com/doi/full/10.1002/tre.857#:~)

35. Slykerman, R.F., et al., 'Effect of *Lactobacillus rhamnosus* HN001 in Pregnancy on Postpartum Symptoms of Depression and Anxiety: A Randomised Double-blind Placebo-controlled Trial', *EBioMedicine*, October 2017 (www.sciencedirect.com/science/article/pii/S2352396417303663)

36. Zidan, Souzan, et al., 'Could psychobiotics and fermented foods improve mood in middle-aged and older women?', *Maturitas*, March 2024 (www.sciencedirect.com/science/article/abs/pii/S0378512223005091#:~)

37. Lee, Chieh-Hsin and Giuliani, Fabrizio, 'The Role of Inflammation in Depression and Fatigue', *Frontiers in*

Immunology, 19 July 2019 (www.ncbi.nlm.nih.gov/pmc/articles/PMC6658985/)

38. Mehdi, Seema, et al., 'Omega-3 Fatty Acids Supplementation in the Treatment of Depression: An Observational Study', *Journal of Personalized Medicine*, 17 January 2023 (www.ncbi.nlm.nih.gov/pmc/articles/PMC9962071/)
39. *Ibid.*
40. Levant, Beth, 'N-3 (*Omega*-3) Fatty Acids in Postpartum Depression: Implications for Prevention and Treatment', *Depression Research and Treatment*, 27 October 2010 (www.ncbi.nlm.nih.gov/pmc/articles/PMC2989696/)
41. Moufidath, Adjibade, et al., 'The Inflammatory Potential of the Diet is Directly Associated with Incident Depressive Symptoms Among French Adults', *The Journal of Nutrition*, July 2019 (www.sciencedirect.com/science/article/pii/S0022316622166605?)
42. Lassale, Camille, et al., 'Healthy dietary indices and risk of depressive outcomes: a systematic review and meta-analysis of observational studies', *Molecular Psychiatry*, 26 September 2018 (www.nature.com/articles/s41380-018-0237-8)
43. Stanford Medicine, 'Stanford Medicine-led study shows why women are at greater risk of autoimmune disease', 1 February 2024 (med.stanford.edu/news/all-news/2024/02/women-autoimmune.html)
44. Iob, Eleonora, et al., 'Adverse childhood experiences and severity levels of inflammation and depression from childhood to young adulthood: a longitudinal cohort study', *Molecular Psychiatry*, 3 March 2022 (www.nature.com/articles/s41380-022-01478-x)
45. Hibbeln, Joseph R., et al., 'Relationships between seafood consumption during pregnancy and childhood and neurocognitive development: Two systematic reviews', University of Bristol, 11 October 2019 (research-information.bris.ac.uk/en/publications/relationships-between-seafood-consumption-during-pregnancy-and-ch)

46. Crawford, Michael A. and Marsh, David E., *The Shrinking Brain* (Filament Publishing, 7 June 2023)
47. Crawford, M. A., et al., 'Evidence for the unique function of docosahexaenoic acid during the evolution of the modern hominid brain', *Lipids*, 1999 (pubmed.ncbi.nlm.nih.gov/10419087/#:~)
48. Jacka, Felice N., et al., 'Western diet is associated with a smaller hippocampus: a longitudinal investigation', *BMC Medicine*, September 2015 (pubmed.ncbi.nlm.nih.gov/26349802/)
49. Yeomans, Martin R., et al., 'Habitual intake of fat and sugar is associated with poorer memory and greater impulsivity in humans', PLoS ONE 18(8): e0290308. 24 August 2023 (journals.plos.org/plosone/article?id=10.1371/journal.pone.0290308)
50. Busch, Morten, 'One quarter of individuals with mental disorder have food addiction', *Science News*, 13 March 2021 (sciencenews.dk/en/one-quarter-of-individuals-with-mental-disorder-have-food-addiction) *and also* Sjogren, Kristian, 'Food addiction is twice as prevalent in adolescents with a mental disorder', *Science News*, 7 May 2023 (sciencenews.dk/en/food-addiction-is-twice-as-prevalent-in-adolescents-with-a-mental-disorder) *and also* Horsager, Christina, et al., 'Food addiction comorbid to mental disorders: A nationwide survey and register-based study', *International Journal of Eating Disorders*, 17 January 2021 (onlinelibrary.wiley.com/doi/10.1002/eat.23472)
51. Bryan, Lucy and Nambisan, Maya, 'Insomnia and Women', Sleep Foundation, 25 March 2024 (www.sleepfoundation.org/insomnia/insomnia-women)
52. Duquenne, Pauline, et al., 'The Association Between Ultra-Processed Food Consumption and Chronic Insomnia in the NutriNet-Santé Study', *Journal of the Academy of Nutrition and Dietetics*, September 2024 (www.jandonline.org/article/S2212-2672(24)00094-7/fulltext)

53. Nutt, David, 'Sleep disorders as core symptoms of depression', *Dialogues in Clinical Neuroscience*, September 2008 (www.ncbi.nlm.nih.gov/pmc/articles/PMC3181883/)
54. Franzen, Peter L., and Buysse, Daniel J., 'Sleep disturbances and depression: risk relationships for subsequent depression and therapeutic implications', *Dialogues in Clinical Neuroscience*, December 2008 (www.ncbi.nlm.nih.gov/pmc/articles/PMC3108260/)
55. Garvan Institute of Medical Research, 'How chronic stress drives the brain to crave comfort food', 8 June 2023 (www.garvan.org.au/news-resources/news/how-chronic-stress-drives-the-brain-to-crave-comfort-food)

Chapter 9. Ageing like fine cheese

1. Women's Health Network, 'Menopause in different cultures', Last Updated: February 27, 2023 (www.womenshealthnetwork.com/menopause-and-perimenopause/menopause-in-different-cultures/)
2. Hickey, Martha, et al., 'Normalising Menopause', *The BMJ*, 15 June 2022 (www.bmj.com/content/377/bmj-2021-069369)
3. Madden, Sharen, et al., 'First Nations women's knowledge of menopause', *CFP*, September 2010 (www.ncbi.nlm.nih.gov/pmc/articles/PMC2939134/)
4. Beyene, Yewoubdar and Martin, Mary C, 'Menopausal Experiences and Bone Density of Mayan Women in Yucatan, Mexico', *American Journal of Human Biology*, 2001 (onlinelibrary.wiley.com/doi/pdf/10.1002/ajhb.1082#:~)
5. Fitzpatrick, K., 'Foraging and Menstruation in the Hadza of Tanzania' , 2018 (https://doi.org/10.17863/CAM.22238)
6. Minkin, Mary Jane, et al., 'Prevalence of postmenopausal symptoms in North America and Europe', *Menopause*, November 2015 (pubmed.ncbi.nlm.nih.gov/25944521/)
7. Blue Zones (www.bluezones.com/explorations/okinawa-japan/#:~), accessed September 2024

8. Nagata, C., et al., 'Soy product intake and hot flashes in Japanese women: results from a community-based prospective study', *American Journal of Epidemiology*, 15 April 2001 (pubmed.ncbi.nlm.nih.gov/11296152/)
9. Bedell, Sarah, et al., 'The pros and cons of plant estrogens for menopause', *The Journal of Steroid Biochemistry and Molecular Biology*, January 2014 (pubmed.ncbi.nlm.nih.gov/23270754/) **and also** Rowe, I. J. and Baber, R. J., *Climacteric*, February 2021 (pubmed.ncbi.nlm.nih.gov/33395316/)
10. CNBC, 'This overlooked corner of women's health could be a $350 billion market opportunity', 15 March 2024 (www.cnbc.com/2024/03/15/this-overlooked-corner-of-womens-health-could-be-a-350-billion-market-opportunity.html)
11. Noll, Priscilla, et al., 'Life habits of postmenopausal women: Association of menopause symptom intensity and food consumption by degree of food processing', *Maturitas*, February 2022 (pubmed.ncbi.nlm.nih.gov/35033227/)
12. Noll, Priscilla, et al., 'Dietary intake and menopausal symptoms in postmenopausal women: a systematic review', *Climacteric*, 2021 (www.tandfonline.com/doi/full/10.1080/13697137.2020.1828854)
13. Herber-Gast, Gerrie-Cor and Mishra, Gita D., 'Fruit, Mediterranean-style, and high-fat and -sugar diets are associated with the risk of night sweats and hot flushes in midlife: results from a prospective cohort study', *The American Journal of Clinical Nutrition*, May 2013 (www.sciencedirect.com/science/article/pii/S0002916523055181?via%3Dihub)
14. Kroenke, Candyce, et al., 'Effects of a dietary intervention and weight change on vasomotor symptoms in the Women's Health Initiative', *Menopause*, September 2012 (journals.lww.com/menopausejournal/abstract/2012/09000/effects_of_a_dietary_intervention_and_weight.8.aspx)

ENDNOTES

15. Soleymani, Mahshid, et al., Dietary patterns and their association with menopausal symptoms: a cross-sectional study', *Menopause*, April 2019 (journals.lww.com/menopausejournal/abstract/2019/04000/dietary_patterns_and_their_association_with.7.aspx)
16. Bermingham, Kate M., et al., 'Menopause is associated with postprandial metabolism, metabolic health and lifestyle: The ZOE PREDICT study', *The Lancet*, November 2022 (www.thelancet.com/journals/ebiom/article/PIIS2352-3964%2822%2900485-6/fulltext)
17. Zoe, 'Davina McCall: Make this choice every day to reduce menopause symptoms', 5 September 2024 (zoe.com/learn/podcast-davina-mccall-menopause)
18. Chen, Zhangling, et al., 'Ultra-Processed Food Consumption and Risk of Type 2 Diabetes: Three Large Prospective U.S. Cohort Studies', *Diabetes Care*, 28 February 2023 (diabetesjournals.org/care/article/46/7/1335/148548/Ultra-Processed-Food-Consumption-and-Risk-of-Type) *and also* Moradi, Sajjad, et al., 'Ultra-Processed Food Consumption and Adult Diabetes Risk: A Systematic Review and Dose-Response Meta-Analysis', *Nutrients*, 9 December 2021 (www.ncbi.nlm.nih.gov/pmc/articles/PMC8705763/) *and also* Grinshpan, Lara Sol, et al., 'Ultra-processed food consumption and non-alcoholic fatty liver disease, metabolic syndrome and insulin resistance: A systematic review', *JHEP Reports*, January 2024 (www.sciencedirect.com/science/article/pii/S2589555923002951) *and also* Srour, Bernard, 'UltraProcessed Food Consumption and Risk of Type 2 Diabetes Among Participants of the NutriNet-Santé Prospective Cohort', *JAMA*, 16 December 2019 (jamanetwork.com/journals/jamainternalmedicine/fullarticle/2757497) *and also* Delpino, Felipe Mendes, et al., 'Ultra-processed food and risk of type 2 diabetes: a systematic review and meta-analysis of longitudinal studies', *International Journal of Epidemiology*, 10 August 2022

(pubmed.ncbi.nlm.nih.gov/34904160/) *and also* Almarshad, Muneerh, et al., 'Relationship between Ultra-Processed Food Consumption and Risk of Diabetes Mellitus: A Mini-Review', *Nutrients*, 7 June 2022 (www.ncbi.nlm.nih.gov/pmc/articles/PMC9228591/)

19. Bhattacharyya, S., et al., 'Exposure to the common food additive carrageenan leads to glucose intolerance, insulin resistance and inhibition of insulin signalling in HepG2 cells and C57BL/6J mice', *Diabetologia*, January 2012 (pubmed.ncbi.nlm.nih.gov/22011715/) *and also* Tobacman, Joanne K., 'Impact of the No-Carrageenan Diet on Glucose Tolerance and Insulin Resistance in Adults with Prediabetes', *Diabetes*, 2018 (diabetesjournals.org/diabetes/article/67/Supplement_1/770-P/58304/Impact-of-the-No-Carrageenan-Diet-on-Glucose)

20. Almarshad, Muneerh, et al., 'Relationship between Ultra-Processed Food Consumption and Risk of Diabetes Mellitus: A Mini-Review', *Nutrients*, 7 June 2022 (www.ncbi.nlm.nih.gov/pmc/articles/PMC9228591/)

21. 'Ultra-processed food and obesity: what is the evidence', Springer Nature, 31 January 2014 (link.springer.com/article/10.1007/s13668-024-00517-z#:~)

22. Lang, Katharine, 'Obesity may increase severity of menopause symptoms, make hormone therapy less effective', *Medical News Today*, 29 September 2023 (www.medicalnewstoday.com/articles/obesity-worsen-menopause-symptoms-reduce-hormone-therapy-efficacy#)

23. Zoe, 'Menopause: Does diet play a part?', 13 March 2023 (zoe.com/learn/podcast-menopause-role-of-diet)

24. TED radio hour. '"Menopause brain" is a real thing. Here's what to do about it', updated 11 November 2022 (www.npr.org/transcripts/973805003)

25. Wilmanski, Tomasz, et al., 'Gut microbiome pattern reflects healthy ageing and predicts survival in humans', *Nature*

metabolism, 18 February 2021 (www.nature.com/articles/s42255-021-00348-0)

26. Peters, Brandilyn A., et al., 'Menopause is Associated with an Altered Gut Microbiome and Estrobolome, with Implications for Adverse Cardiometabolic Risk in the Hispanic Community Health Study/Study of Latinos', 13 April 2022 (journals.asm.org/doi/10.1128/msystems.00273-22)
27. Muhleisen, Alicia L., Herbst-Kralovetz, Melissa M., 'Menopause and the vaginal microbiome', *Maturitas*, September 2016 (pubmed.ncbi.nlm.nih.gov/27451320/) *and also* Dothard, Marisol, 'The effects of hormone replacement therapy on the microbiomes of postmenopausal women', *Climacteric*, April 2023 (www.researchgate.net/publication/369997327_The_effects_of_hormone_replacement_therapy_on_the_microbiomes_of_postmenopausal_women)
28. Peters, Brandilyn A., et al., 'Spotlight on the Gut Microbiome in Menopause: Current Insights', *International Journal of Women's Health*, 10 August 2022 (www.tandfonline.com/doi/full/10.2147/IJWH.S340491)
29. *Ibid.*
30. Odogwu, S., et al., 'Laparoscopic cholecystectomy performed by a surgical care practitioner: a review of outcomes', Royal College of Surgeons, 25 April 2024 (publishing.rcseng.ac.uk/doi/10.1308/rcsann.2023.0058#:~)
31. Unche-Anya, Eugenia, et al., 'Ultraprocessed food consumption and risk of gallstone disease: analysis of 3 prospective cohorts', *The American Journal of Clinical Nutrition*, September 2024 (ajcn.nutrition.org/article/S0002-9165(24)00596-3/abstract)
32. Guts Charity, Gallstones (gutscharity.org.uk/advice-and-information/conditions/gallstones/#:~), accessed September 2024
33. Zaretsky, Janna, et al., 'Ultra-processed food targets bone quality via endochondral ossification', *Bone Research*,

26 February 2021 (www.nature.com/articles/s41413-020-00127-9)

34. Travinsky-Shmul, Tamara, et al., 'Ultra-Processed Food Impairs Bone Quality, Increases Marrow Adiposity and Alters Gut Microbiome in Mice', *Foods*, 15 December 2021 (www.ncbi.nlm.nih.gov/pmc/articles/PMC8701231/)

35. Vogel, Christina, et al., 'Greater access to fast-food outlets is associated with poorer bone health in young children', *Osteoporosis International*, 1 September 2016 (www.ncbi.nlm.nih.gov/pmc/articles/PMC4841385/)

36. Khalid, Nauman, 'Impact of carbonated beverages on early onset of osteoporosis: A narrative review', *Nutrition and Health*, June 2024 (pubmed.ncbi.nlm.nih.gov/37697739/)

37. Tucker, Katherine L., et al., 'Colas, but not other carbonated beverages, are associated with low bone mineral density in older women: The Framingham Osteoporosis Study', *The American Journal of Clinical Nutrition*, October 2006 (www.sciencedirect.com/science/article/pii/S0002916523291170?)

38. Alzheimer's Association, 'Why Does Alzheimer's Disease Affect More Women Than Men? New Alzheimer's Association Grant Will Help Researchers Explore That Question', 11 February 2016 (www.alz.org/blog/alz/february_2016/why_does_alzheimer_s_disease_affect_more_women_tha)

39. Alzheimer's Society, 'Why is the number of people with dementia increasing?', 13 December 2021 (www.alzheimers.org.uk/blog/how-many-people-have-dementia-uk)

40. Alzheimer's Research UK, 'The Impact of Dementia on Women', May 2022 (www.alzheimersresearchuk.org/about-us/our-influence/policy-work/reports/the-impact-of-dementia-on-women/)

41. Alzheimer's Research UK, 'Why Women are bearing more of the impact of dementia', May 2022 (www.alzheimersresearchuk.org/news/why-women-are-bearing-more-of-the-impact-of-dementia/)

42. TED radio hour. '"Menopause brain" is a real thing. Here's what to do about it', updated 11 November 2022 (www.npr.org/transcripts/973805003)
43. Finan, Eileen, 'Everything You Need to Know About Menopausal Brain Fog but Are Afraid to Ask – and No, "You're Not Losing Your Mind"', *People*, 10 March 2024 (people.com/menopausal-brain-fog-lisa-mosconi-the-menopause-brain-exclusive-8605955)
44. Gomes Gonçalves, Natalia, et al., 'Association Between Consumption of Ultraprocessed Foods and Cognitive Decline', *JAMA*, 1 February 2023 (pubmed.ncbi.nlm.nih.gov/36469335/)
45. Li, Huiping, et al., 'Association of Ultraprocessed Food Consumption With Risk of Dementia', *Neurology*, 27 July 2022 (www.neurology.org/doi/10.1212/wnl.0000000000200871)
46. Strour, Bernard, et al., 'Ultra-processed food intake and risk of cardiovascular disease: prospective cohort study (NutriNet-Santé)', *BMJ*, 2019 (www.bmj.com/content/365/bmj.l1451)
47. Robson, David, 'Why the brain's microbiome could hold the key to curing Alzheimer's', *New Scientist*, 19 February 2024 (www.newscientist.com/article/mg26134791-400-why-the-brains-microbiome-could-hold-the-key-to-curing-alzheimers/)
48. Sureda, Antoni, et al., 'Oral microbiota and Alzheimer's disease: Do all roads lead to Rome?', *Pharmacological Research*, January 2020 (www.sciencedirect.com/science/article/abs/pii/S1043661819324831)
49. King's College London, 'Scientists discover links between Alzheimer's disease and gut microbiota', 18 October 2023 (www.kcl.ac.uk/news/links-between-alzheimers-and-gut-microbiota)
50. 'Modulation of Gut Microbiota through dietary intervention in neuroinflammation and Alzheimer's and Parkinson's diseases', *Springer Nature*, 23 April 2024 (link.springer.com/article/10.1007/s13668-024-00539-7) **and also** Edwin

E. Martínez Leo, Edwin E. and Segura Campos, Maira R., 'Effect of ultra-processed diet on gut microbiota and thus its role in neurodegenerative diseases', *Nutrition*, March 2020 (pubmed.ncbi.nlm.nih.gov/31837645/)
51. Dementia UK, 'Young onset dementia: facts and figures' (www.dementiauk.org/information-and-support/young-onset-dementia/young-onset-dementia-facts-and-figures/), accessed September 2024
52. Ahmad, Shafqat, et al., 'Mediterranean Diet Adherence and Risk of All-Cause Mortality in Women', *JAMA*, 31 May 2024 (jamanetwork.com/journals/jamanetworkopen/fullarticle/2819335)
53. Fang, Zhe, et al., 'Association of ultra-processed food consumption with all cause and cause specific mortality: population based cohort study', *BMJ*, 2024 (www.bmj.com/content/385/bmj-2023-078476#:~:)
54. Esposito, Simona, et al., 'Ultra-processed food consumption is associated with the acceleration of biological aging in the Moli-sani Study', *The American Journal of Clinical Nutrition*, December 2024 (www.sciencedirect.com/science/article/abs/pii/S000291652400813X)
55. Blue Zones (www.bluezones.com), accessed September 2024
56. Alonso-Pedrero, Lucia, et al., 'Ultra-processed food consumption and the risk of short telomeres in an elderly population of the Seguimiento Universidad de Navarra (SUN) Project', *American Journal of Clinical Nutrition*, 1 June 2020 (pubmed.ncbi.nlm.nih.gov/32330232/) *and also* Cohut, Maria, 'What are the best foods to fight aging?', *Medical News Today*, 26 January 2018 (www.medicalnewstoday.com/articles/320743)

Chapter 10. A delicious tub of face cream

1. Colour Blind Awareness (www.colourblindawareness.org/colour-blindness), accessed September 2024

ENDNOTES

2. Owen, James, 'Men and Women Really Do See Things Differently', *National Geographic*, 7 September 2012 (www.nationalgeographic.com/culture/article/120907-men-women-see-differently-science-health-vision-sex)
3. Oliveira-Pinto, Ana V., et al., 'Sexual Dimorphism in the Human Olfactory Bulb: Females Have More Neurons and Glial Cells than Males', 5 November 2014 (journals.plos.org/plosone/article?id=10.1371/journal.pone.0111733)
4. Willcox, Kathleen, 'Are Women Better at Tasting Wine Than Men? Science Has the Answer', 13 April 2017, Vinepair (vinepair.com/articles/women-better-tasting-wine-men-science-answer/)
5. Güngör, E. Sönmez, 'Food addiction and gender aspects: Risk factors, co-morbidites and treatment', *European Psychiatry*, 19 July 2023 (www.ncbi.nlm.nih.gov/pmc/articles/PMC10417778/)
6. 'Market size of the flavor and fragrance market worldwide from 2017 to 2023', Statista (www.statista.com/statistics/475081/value-global-flavor-and-fragrance-market/)
7. 'The Top 10 Fragrance Suppliers', *WWD*, 13 October 2005 (wwd.com/feature/the-top-10-fragrance-suppliers-1069385-1827037/)
8. Schlosser, Eric, 'The bitter truth about fast food', *The Guardian*, 7 April 2001 (www.theguardian.com/books/2001/apr/07/features.weekend)
9. Conley, Mikaela, 'Food additive or carcinogen? The growing list of chemicals banned by EU but used in US', *The Guardian*, 23 June 2022 (www.theguardian.com/environment/2022/jun/23/titanium-dioxide-banned-chemicals-carcinogen-eu-us)
10. Inn Express (www.inn-express.com/product-ranges/soft-drinks/diet-pepsi-7l-bib), accessed September 2024
11. Plastic Soup Foundation (www.plasticsoupfoundation.org/en), accessed September 2024

12. Beat the Micro Bead (www.beatthemicrobead.org/get-to-know-microplastics-in-your-cosmetics-part-ii/), accessed September 2024
13. Baulch, Sarah, 'The shocking impacts of plastic pollution in our oceans', Environmental Investigation Agency, 24 May 2013 (eia-international.org/blog/the-shocking-impacts-of-plastic-pollution-in-our-oceans/)
14. 'Forever chemicals in the food aisle' (www.pfasfree.org.uk/wp-content/uploads/Forever-Chemicals-in-the-Food-Aisle-Fidra-2020-.pdf), accessed September 2024
15. 'The sleeping giant of pollution: why the UK must wake up to the impact of toxic chemicals', Wildlife and Countryside (www.wcl.org.uk/assets/uploads/img/files/Chemical_contamination_report_13.06.24.pdf), accessed September 2024
16. '"Forever chemicals" still in use in UK make-up' BBC News, 13 January 2023 (www.bbc.co.uk/news/science-environment-64192516)
17. Edney, Anna, '"Forever Chemicals" Are Still Found in Personal-Care Products', Bloomberg UK, 7 February 2024 (www.bloomberg.com/news/newsletters/2024-02-07/are-pfas-in-skin-care-shampoo-why-forever-chemicals-are-still-everywhere)
18. 'Forever chemicals in the food aisle' (www.pfasfree.org.uk/wp-content/uploads/Forever-Chemicals-in-the-Food-Aisle-Fidra-2020-.pdf), accessed September 2024
19. Boztas, Senay, 'The race to destroy the toxic "forever chemicals" polluting our world', *The Guardian*, 4 January 2024 (www.theguardian.com/environment/2024/jan/04/the-race-to-destroy-the-toxic-forever-chemicals-polluting-our-world)
20. Mamavation, 'PFAs "forever Chemicals" inside sanitary pads and incontinence pads' (www.mamavation.com/beauty/pfas-forever-chemicals-sanitary-pads-incontinence-pads.html) ***and also*** Mamavation, 'Do your tampons contain PFAs "Forever

Chemicals?" They might' (www.mamavation.com/beauty/pfas-tampons.html) *and also* Mamavation, 'Best (& worst) period underwear & period panties tested for indications of PFAs' (www.mamavation.com/health/period-underwear-contaminated-pfas-chemicals.html), accessed September 2024

21. Marroquin, Joanna, et al., 'Chemicals in menstrual products: A systematic review', *BJOG*, April 2024 (pubmed.ncbi.nlm.nih.gov/37743685/)
22. Gao, Chong-Jing and Kannan, Kurunthachalam, 'Phthalates, bisphenols, parabens, and triclocarban in feminine hygiene products from the United States and their implications for human exposure', *Environmental International*, March 2020 (www.sciencedirect.com/science/article/pii/S0160412019333859)
23. Park, Chan Jin, et al., 'Sanitary pads and diapers contain higher phthalate contents than those in common commercial plastic products', *Reproductive Toxicology*, March 2019 (www.sciencedirect.com/science/article/abs/pii/S0890623818302259?via%3Dihub)
24. Endocrine Society, 'Phthalate exposure may increase diabetes risk in women' (www.endocrine.org/news-and-advocacy/news-room/2023/phthalate-exposure-may-increase-diabetes-risk-in-women)
25. Nobles, Carrie J., et al., 'Preconception Phthalate Exposure and Women's Reproductive Health: Pregnancy, Pregnancy Loss, and Underlying Mechanisms', *Environmental Health Perspective*, December 2023 (pubmed.ncbi.nlm.nih.gov/38088888/)
26. Basso, Carla Giovana, et al., 'Exposure to phthalates and female reproductive health: A literature review', *Reproductive Toxicology*, April 2022 (www.sciencedirect.com/science/article/abs/pii/S0890623822000260)
27. Zota, Ami R., et al., 'Temporal Trends in Phthalate Exposures: Findings from the National Health and Nutrition Examination Survey, 2001–2010', *Environmental*

28. Clements, Barbara, 'Pregnant women should avoid ultraprocessed, fast foods', University of Washington Medicine, 6 February 2024 (https://newsroom.uw.edu/news-releases/study-pregnant-women-should-avoid-ultraprocessed-fast-foods)
29. Ibid.
30. Zota, Ami R. and Shamasunder, Bhavna, 'The Environmental Injustice of Beauty: Framing Chemical Exposures from Beauty Products as a Health Disparities Concern', *American Journal of Obstetrics & Gynecology*, 6 February 2024 (www.ncbi.nlm.nih.gov/pmc/articles/PMC5614862/)
31. Ibid.
32. FDA, 'Phthalates in Cosmetics', last updated May 19, 2022 (www.fda.gov/cosmetics/cosmetic-ingredients/phthalates-cosmetics#cos)
33. Chaichiam, Shahla, et al., 'Toxicological impact of Bisphenol A on females' reproductive system: Review based on experimental and epidemiological studies', *Springer Nature*, 26 March 2024 (link.springer.com/article/10.1007/s43032-024-01521-y#:~)
34. Pivonello, Claudia, et al., 'Bisphenol A: an emerging threat to female fertility', Reproductive Biology and Endocrinology, 14 March 202 (rbej.biomedcentral.com/articles/10.1186/s12958-019-0558-8)
35. 'BPA Exposure of the Placenta Could Affect Fetal Brain Development', *Neuroscience*, 12 January 2022 (neurosciencenews.com/bpa-fetal-development-19902/)
36. Hatch, Cory, 'BPA in pregnancy linked to behavior problems in baby girls', NBC News, 24 October 2011 (www.nbcnews.com/health/health-news/bpa-pregnancy-linked-behavior-problems-baby-girls-flna1c9453689) *and also* Exposure to chemical BPA before birth linked to behavioral, emotional difficulties in girls', Harvard School of Public

Health, 24 October 2011 (https://www.sciencedaily.com/releases/2011/10/111024084637.htm)
37. Swan, Shanna S., *Count Down: How Our Modern World Is Threatening Sperm Counts, Altering Male and Female Reproductive Development, and Imperiling the Future of the Human Race* (Scribner, 2021)
38. Gao, Chong-Jing and Kannan, Kurunthachalam, 'Phthalates, bisphenols, parabens, and triclocarban in feminine hygiene products from the United States and their implications for human exposure', *Environment International*, March 2020 (www.sciencedirect.com/science/article/pii/S0160412019333859)
39. Cancer Research, UK, 'Can cosmetics cause cancer?' (www.cancerresearchuk.org/about-cancer/causes-of-cancer/cancer-myths/cosmetics), accessed September 2024
40. Breast Cancer UK, 'Chemicals and environment: Endocrine system and EDCs' (www.breastcanceruk.org.uk/reduce-your-risk/chemicals-and-our-environment/endocrine-system-and-edcs/), accessed September 2024
41. Soil Association, 'What are the benefits of using organic beauty and wellbeing products?' (www.soilassociation.org/take-action/organic-living/beauty-wellbeing/why-choose-organic-beauty/), accessed September 2024
42. EU Environment (environment.ec.europa.eu/topics/circular-economy/eu-ecolabel_en), accessed September 2024
43. Women's Voices For the Earth, 'Unpacking the Fragrance Industry: Policy Failures, the Trade Secret Myth and Public Health', updated September 2018 (https://womensvoices.org/wp-content/uploads/2018/09/Fragrance_Report_Updates_2018.pdf)

Chapter 11. Disrespecting the Mother

1. The Big Plastic Count, 'The Big Plastic Count Results Are In!' (thebigplasticcount.com/results), accessed September 2024

2. United Nations Development Program 'Why aren't we recycling more plastic?', 28 November 2023 (stories.undp.org/why-arent-we-recycling-more-plastic)
3. UK Parliament, Plastic Waste, 20 March 2024 (commonslibrary.parliament.uk/research-briefings/cbp-8515/)
4. Cowger, Win, et al., 'Global producer responsibility for plastic pollution', *Science Advances*, 24 April 2024 (www.science.org/doi/10.1126/sciadv.adj8275#sec-2)
5. Morunga, Aden Miles, 'Unbottling the truth: Coca Cola's role in plastic pollution', Greenpeace, 26 September 2023 (www.greenpeace.org/aotearoa/story/unbottling-the-truth-coca-colas-role-in-plastic-pollution/)
6. Bite Back, 'Research Unearths How Big Food Impacts Planetary Health', 18 September 2024 (www.biteback2030.com/our-activists/stories/research-reveals-how-big-food-digs-into-planetary-health/)
7. Tillack, Gemma, 'Why "Roundtable on Sustainable Palm Oil (RSPO)" palm oil is neither responsible nor sustainable', Rainforest Action Network, 25 April 2013 (www.ran.org/the-understory/why_rspo_sustainable_palm_oil_is_not_responsible/)
8. Human Rights Watch '"When We Lost the Forest, We Lost Everything": Oil Palm Plantations and Rights Violations in Indonesia', 22 September 2019 (www.hrw.org/report/2019/09/23/when-we-lost-forest-we-lost-everything/oil-palm-plantations-and-rights-violations)
9. Niko, Nikodemus, et al., 'Indigenous Women's Connection to Forest: Colonialism, Lack of Land Ownership and Livelihood Deprivations of Dayak Benawan in Indonesia', *Feminist Encounters: A Journal of Critical Studies in Culture and Politics*, 1 March 2024 (www.lectitopublishing.nl/download/indigenous-womens-connection-to-forest-colonialism-lack-of-land-ownership-and-livelihood-14233.pdf)

10. Benazir, Citra, 'The perilous life of female palm oil plantation workers in Papua', Palmoil.io, 18 April 2023 (blog.palmoil.io/female-palm-oil-plantation-worker-in-papua/)
11. Oxfam, 'Behind the brands: Food justice and the "Big 10" food and beverage companies', 26 February 2013 (www-cdn.oxfam.org/s3fs-public/file_attachments/bp166-behind-the-brands-260213-en_2.pdf)
12. World Worldlife Fund, Palm Oil (wwf.panda.org/discover/our_focus/food_practice/sustainable_production/palm_oil/), accessed September 2024
13. George, Richard, '5 problems with "sustainable" palm oil', Greenpeace, 1 November 2019 (www.greenpeace.org.uk/news/5-problems-with-sustainable-palm-oil/)
14. Tillack, Gemma, 'Why "Roundtable on Sustainable Palm Oil (RSPO)" palm oil is neither responsible nor sustainable', Rainforest Action Network, 25 April 2013 (www.ran.org/the-understory/why_rspo_sustainable_palm_oil_is_not_responsible/)
15. Waring, Louisianna, 'Soya's deadly secret', *The Ecologist*, 6 February 2020 (theecologist.org/2020/feb/06/soyas-deadly-secret)
16. World Worldlife Fund, Soy (wwf.panda.org/discover/our_focus/food_practice/sustainable_production/soy/), accessed September 2024
17. 'Deforestation surges in Brazil's sensitive Cerrado region', *Financial Times*, 14 January 2024 (www.ft.com/content/3156a1f8-8b9e-4ae3-b77c-53d293d72f4c)
18. Skidmore, Marin Elizabeth, et al., 'Agricultural intensification and childhood cancer in Brazil', *PNAS*, 30 October 2023 (www.pnas.org/doi/full/10.1073/pnas.2306003120)
19. Lambert, Jonathan, 'Growing Corn Is A Major Contributor To Air Pollution, Study Finds', *The Salt*, 1 April 2019 (www.npr.org/sections/thesalt/2019/04/01/708818581/growing-corn-is-a-major-contributor-to-air-pollution-study-finds)

20. National Oceanic and Atmospheric Association, 'Gulf of Mexico "dead zone" is the largest ever measured', National Ocean Service website, 2 August 2017 (www.noaa.gov/media-release/gulf-of-mexico-dead-zone-is-largest-ever-measured)
21. Harvey, Fiona, 'Dust bowl conditions of 1930s US now more than twice as likely to reoccur', *The Guardian*, 18 May 2020 (www.theguardian.com/environment/2020/may/18/us-dust-bowl-conditions-likely-to-reoccur-great-plains)
22. Feedback, 'Too much of a bad thing: The use and misuse of IUK soil and land to grow sugar', December 2019 (feedbackglobal.org/wp-content/uploads/2019/11/Too-much-of-a-bad-thing-the-use-and-misuse-of-land-and-soils-to-grow-sugar-Feedback-2019.pdf)
23. Soil Association, 'Ultra-Processed Planet' (www.soilassociation.org/media/23032/soilassociation_upf_2023_digital.pdf), accessed September 2024
24. Cosier, Susan, 'The world needs topsoil to grow 95% of its food – but it's rapidly disappearing', *The Guardian*, 30 May 2019 (www.theguardian.com/us-news/2019/may/30/topsoil-farming-agriculture-food-toxic-america)
25. National Academies Committee, *Exploring Linkages Between Soil Health and Human Health*, National Academies Press, 2024 (nap.nationalacademies.org/read/27459/chapter/2#10)
26. Brown, Marina D., et al., 'Fecal and soil microbiota composition of gardening and non-gardening families', *Scientific Reports*, 31 January 2022 (pubmed.ncbi.nlm.nih.gov/35102166/)
27. Roslund, Marja I., et al., 'Scoping review on soil microbiome and gut health – Are soil microorganisms missing from the planetary health plate?', British Ecological Society, 24 April 2024 (besjournals.onlinelibrary.wiley.com/doi/10.1002/pan3.10638)
28. Huebl, Lena, et al., 'Geophagy in Northern Uganda: Perspectives from Consumers and Clinicians', *The American*

Journal of Tropical Medicine and Hygiene, December 2016 (www.ncbi.nlm.nih.gov/pmc/articles/PMC5154465/#:~)

29. Liddicoat, Craig, et al., 'Naturally-diverse airborne environmental microbial exposures modulate the gut microbiome and may provide anxiolytic benefits in mice', *Science of the Total Environment*, 28 October 2019 (pubmed.ncbi.nlm.nih.gov/31704402/)

30. Faleiros, Gustavo and Andreoni, Manuela, 'Agro-suicide: Amazon deforestation hits Brazil's soy producers', Dialogue Earth, 15 October 2020 (dialogue.earth/en/food/37887-agri-suicide-amazon-deforestation-hits-rain-brazils-soy-producers/)

31. Quaglia, Sofia 'Survey finds that 60 firms are responsible for half of world's plastic pollution', *The Guardian*, 24 April 2024 (www.theguardian.com/environment/2024/apr/24/survey-finds-that-60-firms-are-responsible-for-half-of-worlds-plastic-pollution)

32. Gustavsson, Jenney, et al., Food and Agriculture Organization of the United Nations, 'Global Food Losses and Food Waste', Food and Agriculture Organization of the United Nations, 2011 (www.fao.org/4/mb060e/mb060e.pdf)

33. 'Livestock and landscapes', Food and Agriculture Organization of the United Nations, 2012 (openknowledge.fao.org/server/api/core/bitstreams/c93da831-30b3-41dc-9e12-e1ae2963abde/content), accessed September 2024

34. IDDRI Study, 'An agroecological Europe in 2050: multifunctional agriculture for healthy eating', 18 September 2018 (www.soilassociation.org/media/18074/iddri-study-tyfa.pdf)

Chapter 12. Seeds of Change

1. Nickerson, Kourtney P., et al., 'Deregulation of intestinal anti-microbial defense by the dietary additive, maltodextrin', *Gut Microbes*, 4 March 2015 (www.ncbi.nlm.nih.gov/pmc/articles/PMC4615306/) ***and also*** Zangara, Megan T, et al.,

'Maltodextrin Consumption Impairs the Intestinal Mucus Barrier and Accelerates Colitis Through Direct Actions on the Epithelium', *Frontiers in Immunology*, 14 March 2022 (www.ncbi.nlm.nih.gov/pmc/articles/PMC8963984/)
2. O'Hare, Ryan, 'Plant-based UPFs linked with higher risk of cardiovascular disease', Imperial News, 11 June 2024 (www.imperial.ac.uk/news/254034/plant-based-upfs-linked-with-higher-risk/)

Index

Note: page numbers in bold refer to **diagrams**, page numbers in *italics* refer to information contained in tables.

Abbott 78
Abrams–Rivera, Carlos 115
Academy of Nutrition and Dietetics (AND) 69, 77–9
Adam 140, 229
addiction 98, 110–11, 113, 116, 182–3, 193, 256
adolescents 93, 94, 140
adverse childhood experiences (ACEs) 168, 177
adverse pregnancy outcomes (APOs) 132
advertising 63–73, 84–6, 91–3, 95, 113–16
Advertising Standards Authority 71
ageing 185–210
agro-suicide 247
agroecology 244
agroforestry 245
alcoholic drinks 33–4, 95, 196, 203, 209, 299
alcopops 34, 299
Allen, Lily 60
almond 46
Altria 232
Alzheimer's disease 43, 106–7, 204–7
Amazon rainforest 236, 238–9
American Beverage Association 68, 69
American Dietetic Association (ADA) 77
American Society of Nutrition 80
ancestors 142, 178
anchoring 294
Ancient Egyptians 166

animal feed 235, 240
anogenital distance (AGD) 159, 221
anorexia 72, 76
anti-inflammatory diets 146, 153, 177–8, 184
antibiotics 126
antidepressants 165, 177
anxiety 42, 72, 88, 90–1, 94, 109, 174
   and body weight 98
   and the gut microbiome 128, 130–1
   and Premenstrual Dysphoric Disorder 179
   and psychobiotics 175–6
   and UPFs 170, 171, 175
appetite 102
   regulation 108, 180
   suppression 41, 112–13
apples 42, 44–7, 101, 108–10, 151, 184, 297
Aptamil 82, 83, 87–9
Aquinas, Thomas 166
archetypes, feminine 62, 64, 230
Aristotle 166
arthritis 133, 154
artificial sweeteners 24, 68, 70, 153–4, 170–1, 174, 195
aspartame 68, 70, 153–4, 170–1
asthma 3, 122, 160
Attenborough, David 233
Aunt Jemima 66, 67

autoimmune conditions 3, 4, 120, 151–5
aviation industry 232

babies, microbiome 121–3, 133
bacon 295–6
bacteria
   therapeutic use 175–6
   see also gut microbiome
bacterial vaginosis (BV) 126
'bad foods' 41, 76–8, 80–1, 96, 265
baked beans 31
bakery aisles 28–9
balanced diets 104, 197, 203
   'everything is fine as part of a balanced diet' message 78–81
barbeques 69
batch-cooking 300–1
bean(s)
   broccoli and white bean soup 270
   spicy bean soup 269–70
beef 236
beer 33, 299
befriending 172
Bernays, Edward 64–5
Best (magazine) 117, 121
Betty Crocker 28, 64, 64–8, 73, 74
Big Food 4–5, 104, 115, 260
big industry, as cause of damage to human health 94–5, 98

INDEX

binge-eating disorder 110, 111, 179
bipolar disorder 174
Birds Eye 101–2
biscuits 22, 24, 28, 92, 108, 200–1, 241, 256, 294
   homemade 275–6
Bisphenol A (BPA) 222–4
Bite Back 232
black people 66–8
blood pressure 54, 105, 157
blood sugar 46–7, 93, 102, 194–5, 198, 265, 298
blood-brain barrier (BBB) 174, 181
'Blue Zones' 208, 299
body *see* female body; male body
body fat 93, 97, 100–1
   active 105
   distribution 194
   and menarche 143
body mass index (BMI) 54, 93, 104, 106, 170
   average American 99
   high 106
   and menarche 142–4
   and menopause 191, 193, 195–6
body positivity 71
body-mind connection 164–5
bones 142, 202–4
borderline personality disorder (BPD) 129–30
Boycott, Rosie 61

brain 94, 108–9, 174, 179–83
   blood flow 207
   and cognitive decline 205–7
   and fish 178
   inflammation 177
   reward centre 108–9, 110–11, 179–80
   see also gut-brain axis
brain fog 205
brain microbiome 207
branding 67
Brazil 236–40, 247
bread 277–80, 301
   artisan 25
   French 28–9, 53
   homemade 25, 277–80
   sourdough 28, 277–9
   supermarket 21, 24, 278–9
   ultra-processed 21, 24, 28–9
   wraps (recipe) 280
breakfast cereals 24, 32, 261–2, 301
breakfasts 188, 261–4
breast cancer 105–6, 143, 204, 225
breast milk 81, 83–4, 90, 222
breastfeeding 76, 81–90, 243
   support for 86–8
Briden, Lara 194
brioche 29
British Broadcasting Corporation (BBC) 156, 220, 239
British Journal of Midwifery 88–9

British Medical Journal 5, 42, 94, 171
British Nutrition Foundation (BNF) 79–80, 114
British Sugar 114, 241
broccoli and white bean soup 270
bulimia 111, 179
butter 293

Cadbury's 110
   Dairy Milk 30–1, 114
   Smash 51, 52
caesarean section 118, 121–2, 156
cake mixes 64–5
cakes 24, 28, 200–1, 294, 297
   homemade 274–5
calcium 203–4
calorie intake 41, 72
calorie restriction 72
calorie-dense foods 102, 256
Campaign Against Living Miserably (CALM) 167
Canadian Sugar Institute 69
cancer 39, 42, 104, 113, 143, 204, 208, 225, 237
   female 43, 105–6, 124, 126–8
candida albicans 125
capitalism 61, 74
carb to fat ratio 109–10, *109*
carbon capture 250
carbon dioxide emissions 232
carcinogens 68, 171, 217

cardiovascular disease 42, 93, 103, 154, 195, 295
carers 205
Carne, Kirsty 203–4
carrageenan 216
celebrity chefs, gender bias 49
cereal snack bars 24, 30, 45–6
cerebrovascular disease 207
Cerrado 236–8
cervical cancer 126
Chan, Andrew 170
change 248, **251**, 253–302, 305–7
charities 114
cheese 11, 23, 27, 283–5, 297
   grated 27
   vegan 294, 295
chelating agents 31–2, 216
chicha (fermented drink) 237–8
Child, Julia 68
childbirth 117–18, 121–2, 155–8
childcare, women and 61
childhood obesity 93, 99
childhood sexual abuse 111, 177
childhood trauma/abuse 111, 129–30, 168, 177
children 13, 75–96
   as customers for life 91–3
   and packed lunches 272–3
   proportion of UPFs consumed by 92
chilled food aisle 27
chocolate 30–1

INDEX

cholecystectomy 200–2
cholesterol levels 70, 94
chorizo 295–6
Christianity 166, 238
chromosomes 151–2, 177, 209, 212–13
chronic disease 94–5, 198
   see also non-communicable diseases
cider 33
climate change 39
Clinton, Hilary 60
Coca-Cola 44, 68–9, 78–9, 95, 114, 232, 239, 247
'cocktail effect' 225
coconut milk 23, 253
coeliac disease 154–5
cognitive decline 205–7
Coke Zero 70
colour vision 212–13
comfort eating 108–9, 111, 183–4
Cominesi, Cynthia Moleta 238–9, 243
commerciogenic malnutrition (baby bottle disease) 85
Conagra 67
condiments 31–2, 288–90
consumption 9, 218, 226
contraceptive pill 145, 147
cookies, homemade 275–6
cooking 51–2
   men and 49

UPF's denigration of 7, 12–13, 51, 57, 59–60, 63–4, 74, 307
   women and 6–7, 12–13
corn crops 237, 239–41, 244
cortisol 174, 196
cosmetics 211–12, 214, 215–27
Costa 79
couscous 31
Covid-19 pandemic 9, 89, 192, 204, 214
cows 240
cow's milk 27, 86
crackers, easy 267
cravings 98, 102, 193, 197
Crawford, Michael 178
cream cheese 23, 27
creation mythology 140, 229–30
Cree people 10
crisps 22, 39–40, 92, 102, 253–4, 266, 273, 301
critical thinking 96
Crohn's disease 153
crumble, fruit 297
cupcakes, simple 274–5
cured meats 27
custard, ultra-processed 23
Cyrus, Miley 60

da Silva, Lula 236
dairy 27
   see also butter; cheese; yoghurt
Danone 44, 79, 80, 82, 89, 232

DATEM 29, 45
Davidson, Terry 180–2
Dayak Benawen people 234
dead zones 240
death 42–3, 95
deforestation 233–6, 247
dementia 43, 106–7, 204–8
dental health 94, 174
depression 3–4, 43, 107, 109, 163–84
   and inflammation 176–8, 183
   and the microbiome 128, 130–1, 133, 199
   post-natal 171, 175
   and psychobiotics 175–6
   risk factors 170
desserts 296–7
Devil 166
DEXA scans 202
diabetes 93, 104, 221
   gestational 105, 157, 158
   Type 2 39, 42–3, 47, 54, 103, 122, 195, 198
Diagnostic and Statistical Manual of Mental Disorders (DSM) 167
Diet Coke 70, 184
'diet' foods 70–1
diet industry 112
dietary support 172–3
dieticians 4–5, 68–9
dieting 112–15, 193–4
dimethicone (E900) 217–18, 219

Dinan, Ted 176
Diwali 10
docosahexaenoic acid (DHA) 176, 178
dog food 303–4, 307–8
Dolmio 50, 59
domestic chores 73
dopamine 108–11, 170, 173, 179–80
Douglas, Michael 8
dressings 289–90
dry ingredients aisle 31–2
Duncan, Helen 192–4

E442 31
E476 31
eating
   compulsive 109
   emotion-related 108–10, 182
   healthy 50, 72–3, 78, 94, 207–8
   mindful 73
   mindless 113
   overeating 108–9, 183–4
   speed of 41
eating disorders 71–2, 76, 110–11, 179
eating out 299–300
'eating your environment' approach 56
eczema 122
EDTA 31–2, 216, 288
eggs 262–3, 288–9
   'Add an Egg' concept 63–5

emotion-related eating 108–10, 182
emotions 13, 98
emulsifiers 31, 45, 103, 153, 174
endocrine disrupting chemicals (EDCs) 142, 221, 223–5
endometrial cancer 127–8
endometrial microbiome 127, 131–2
endometriosis 106, 124, 127–8, 144, 148, 150, 161, 222
energy drinks 34, 143, 298
environment
   'eating your environment' approach 56
   gene-environment interaction 152–3
   impact of the UPF industry upon 230–41, 243–4, 247–8
Environmental Investigation Agency 219
environmentalists 77
Esquire (magazine) 39
ethics, profits over 84–90
EU Ecolabel 227
European Union (EU), regulations 30
Eve 140
evening meals 280–5
evolution 55, 152, 213–14, 245
exploitation 75–96, 230–1, 234, 243, 250

farming
   intensive 240, 241, 242, 248, 249
   'no-till' 238, 243
   organic 249–50
   regenerative 243–7
fast foods 67, 93, 95–6, 143, 147, 150, 203, 268, 300–1
fat, body *see* body fat
'fat free' 70, 71
fathers, absent 142
fats, dietary 19
   carb to fat ratio 109–10, *109*
   and the food matrix 46
   hydrogenated 70–1, 127
   saturated 180–1, 191
   trans 70–1, 127, 150, 233
   UPF content 24, 40–1, 100–1, 109–10, *109*
   see also high fat diets/foods; 'low fat' products; omega-3 fatty acids; omega-6 fatty acids
Fávaro, Carlos 236–7
Fazzino, Tera 101–2
Fe-Fi-Fo study 134
'fed is best' message 81–4, 90
female body 139–41
   as faulty 2, 140–1, 161
   impact of UPFs on 43
   shame regarding 139–40
female emancipation 65
female empowerment 60
female professions 68–9

female subjugation 62
feminine hygiene products 221, 225, 227
feminists 60, 61, 88
fermented foods 55–6, 134–8, 175, 198, 200, 236–8
Ferrero 44
fertility 2–3, 13, 105, 127, 132, 139, 148–51, 159, 222–3
fibre 16, 40, 100–1, 103, 125, 127–8, 134, 143, 146, 150, 170, 178, 242
   and the menopause 188, 191, 199–200
   and the microbiome 103, 121, 123, 125, 127–8, 134, 173–4, 184, 188
fibroids 127, 128
fibromyalgia 153–4
Fidra 220
First Steps Nutrition Trust 86, 91
fish 26, 176–7, 178
   oily 94, 177, 184, 198, 292–3
fizzy drinks 3, 34, 67–8, 70, 93, 113, 143, 147, 159–60, 184, 198, 203, 248, 298, 301
flavour, UPF-free 286–7
flavourings 24, 215
Floyd, George 66
focus, lack of 9
Follow-on Milks 86
food
   colour 212–14

   foraged 54–5, 56
   mindful approach to 10, 13, 25, 57, 73
   pleasure of 76–7
   single-ingredient 257–8
   see also processed food; *specific foods*; ultra-processed food
Food & Drug Administration (FDA) 220
food addiction 98, 110–11, 113, 116, 182–3, 193, 256
food additives 4, 77, 92, 103, 195, 256
   and autoimmune conditions 155
   and the microbiome 121, 132
   and pregnancy 132
   see also specific additives
food allergies 48, 91, 294, 295
food cues 181
'Food Day' 1975 38
food fear 72
food guilt 72
food industry 104
   and gender imbalance 7
   influence 4–5, 38, 78–80, 88–9, 114
   male CEOs of 49, 115
   profit-focus 4, 17, 25, 44–5, 247, 307
food labels 4, 48, 217, 248, 292
   clean labelling 4

food industry's influence
on 5
Nova 4 classification
examples 21–3
food matrix 45–7, 102, 110,
121, 298
food relationship 13, 25, 76–7,
98, 212
women's toxic 97–116
food shopping 10–12, 47–8, 51,
73, 257–9
local 260–1
food waste 10
foods, wild 54–6
foraged foods 54–5, 56
Foreign Service 61
formula milks 78, 81–90, 95,
120
fossil fuels 95, 232
fragrance 215, 227
'free from' products 294–5
freedom of choice 80, 83,
89–90, 115
French cuisine 28–9, 51–4, 56,
68
Freud, Sigmund 64–5, 167
frozen foods 32–3, 48, 50–1,
257
fruit 26, 297
fruit crumble 297
fruit juices 46–7, 298

gallbladder problems 200–2
gender inequality 6–7, 13, 60,
73–4

gender knowledge gap 139
gender roles, traditional 7, 12,
59–74
gene-environment interaction
152–3
General Mills 64–5, 67–8, 78
Gerber, Daniel 62–3, 70
Gerber, Dorothy 63
Geréb, Ágnes 117
ghrelin 41
Givaudan 215
global warming 236
GLP-1 agonists 182
glucose-fructose syrup 241
glycogen 125, 126
Go Ahead bars 22, 45, 113
God 140, 229–30, 238
'good food' 41
government 108, 114
gratitude 10, 13, 25, 57
Great Plains 241
Green, Nancy 66
Greenland 55–6
Greenpeace 235
greenwashing 247
Greer, Germaine 139
Greggs PLC 79, 114
Guarani-Kaiowá community
236–8
Guardian (newspaper) 61
Gussow, Joan Dye 38
gut dysbiosis 154
gut microbiome 94, 102–3,
117–38, 146, 150, 184

and autoimmune disorders
   154
 boosting 54, 56
 and dementia 207
 and the menopause 187–9,
   199
 and mental health 170,
   173–5
 and soil microbes 242–2
gut-brain axis 119, 128–31,
   163, 174, 176

Hadza people 186
Haines, Jane 179
Hall, Kevin 39–42, 49–50, 100
ham 295–6
hanger 164
Harman, Toni 117–18, 121–2,
   133
Harper, Joyce 190
health 74, 93, 98, 140–1
   at risk nature of 13
   impact of diet on 1
   impact of UPFs on 2–4, 13,
     35, 39–40, 42–4, 103–4
   and the menopause 195–6
   and obesity 99, 105–7
   sidelining of women's
     189–90
   and smoking 116
   and unprocessed diets 54–7
   vital signs of 145
'health by association'
   messaging 114
health claims 70–1, 261–2

Health Survey for England
   98–9
healthy eating 50, 72–3, 78, 94,
   207–8
heart disease 39, 42–3, 70, 93,
   104, 133, 198, 208
high fat diets/foods 111, 126,
   147, 170, 179–81, 191, 193,
   195, 198, 202–3
high sugar diets/foods 111, 126,
   147, 150, 170, 179–81, 183,
   191, 193–5, 202–3
high-fat-high-carb foods 111
high-fructose corn syrup
   (HFCS) 239, 241
Hilton, Paris 118
hippocampus 180–2, 207
Hippocrates 166
Hispanic people 67
hormonal imbalances 145
hormone-replacement therapy
   (HRT) 3, 125, 185, 188–90,
   195–6, 199
Horton, Kate 201–2
hot flushes 186, 188, 191,
   195–6, 208
Human Papillomavirus (HPV)
   126–7
Human Rights Watch 234
hummus, easy 266
hunger 41, 102
hunter-gatherers 120, 186, 213
hunters 10
hydrogenated fats 70–1, 127

INDEX

hyperpalatability 16, 17, 41–2, 101–2, 105, 110, 213, 256
hysteria 166–7

ice cream 20, 32–3, 70, 98, 109, 113, 216, 241, 254, 294, 297, 301
Iceland 233
Ikaria, Greece 208
immune system 151–2, 154, 174, 177
indigenous people 9–10, 12, 55–6, 186, 219, 229–30, 234, 236–8, 244
Indonesia 234, 263
Infant Feeding Survey 87
inflammation 103, 105, 133–4, 154, 176–7, 207
   chronic 170, 177
   and dementia 207
   and depression 176–8
   'fast-food fever' 145–6
   and the menopause 198
   and omega-6 fatty acids 291–2
   see also anti-inflammatory diets
Inflammatory Bowel Disease (IBD) 153
influencers 4–5, 68, 72
ingredients, checking 226
insomnia 183, 205
Instagram 5, 68, 72
insulin resistance 194–7
Intelligence Quotient (IQ) 178

interconnectedness 10, 248, 306
International Flavours and Fragrances (IFF) 215
Inuit diet 55–6
irritable bowel syndrome (IBS) 120

Japan 186, 187, 208
junk food 24–5, 38, 78, 93, 146

Keely, Alice 157–8
Keen, Mike 55–6
kefir 135, 137
Kellogg's 44, 78, 79, 216, 262
Kendamil 88–9
Kentucky Fried Chicken (KFC) 59, 111, 114
ketchup 31, 288
kimchi 135, 136–7, 138
Kimmerer, Robin Wall 244
kisspeptin 143
kitchen equipment 259–60
kitchen stereotypes 59–74
Koistinen, Ina Schuppe 123, 161
kombucha 134–5
Kraft 44, 101–2
Kraft Heinz 44, 114–15

lacto-fermentation 135–6
lactobacillus 123, 124–7, 175
lateral habenula 183
Lawson, Nigella 60
Lee, James 153

leptin 103, 143
Lerner, Aaron 154–5
libido 150–1, 184, 195
lignan 188
longevity 175, 187, 207–8
'low calorie' products 70, 71
'low fat' products 5, 16, 70–1
'low sugar' diets 125, 147
Lunchables 101–2
lunches 92, 114–15, 267–8, 272–3
Lupus 4, 120, 151
Lynn, Helen 225–6

McDonald's 79, 114, 136, 201, 253
Maggi, Blairo 236
maize 237, 239–41, 244
male body, as default 139
male 'people', as default human 1
male privilege 139–40
malnutrition 87–8
maltodextrin 216, 271
Mammy stereotype 66–7
margarine 293
'Marriage Bar' 61
Mars 5, 44, 80, 114, 307
maternal microbiome 130, 131–3
maternal nutrition 178
matrescence 140
Matthias, Torsten 154–5
mayo, easy (recipe) 288–9
mealtimes 13, 51–2, 96, 258–9

meat 10
  coated/marinated 26
  cured 27, 295–6
  dried 27
  grass-fed 249
  minimally processed 26
  organic 249
  processed 147, 149, 190, 295–6
  red 127, 149, 296
meat glue 95, 154–5
meat-free products 217, 294, 295
Mediterranean-style diet 3, 115, 143, 146, 150, 171–2, 190–1, 205–6, 208
memory 180–2, 207
men
  and cooking 6–7, 69
  food marketed at 69–70
  and obesity 99
  see also male...
menarche 140, 141–4
menopause 2, 3, 43, 130, 140, 161, 185–200
  and body weight 191–4
  and dementia 205
  and lifestyle change 196–7
  as lucrative market 189–90
  medicalization 185
  and mental health 175–6
  and obesity 105–6
  in other cultures 185–6, 189
  and probiotics 134
  as upgrade 186–7

INDEX

what to eat during 197–8
menstrual cycle 2, 105, 130, 145–6, 168
menstrual products 221, 227
menstruation 144–8, 161
  and cultural messaging 140
  as fifth vital sign 145
  heavy (menorrhagia) 2–3, 43, 144–6
  onset 140, 141–4
  painful (dysmenorrhea) 2–3, 43, 144–6
mental health 42, 94, 107, 129–30, 163–84, 199
  see also anxiety; depression
'mental load' 4
menu planning 47–8
metabolic health 46–7, 196
metformin 147
methyl cellulose 217
mice studies 170–1, 183, 203, 243
  gender bias 130, 139–40, 152, 170
microbes 13
microbiome 54, 56, 94, 102–3, 117–38, 305
  brain 207
  depletion 120–1
  endometrial 127, 131–2
  and fibre 103, 121, 123, 125, 127–8, 134, 173–4, 184, 188
  and insomnia 183
  maternal 130, 131–3
  and the menopause 199
  and puberty onset 143
  seeding 121–3
  vaginal 121–7, 137, 150, 161
  see also gut microbiome
microbirthing 121–3
microgenderome 119–20
microplastics 149, 218–19
microsexome 119–20
milk 30–1
  cow's 27, 86
  plant-based 254, 295
'milk nurses' 84–5
mindful approach to food 10, 13, 25, 57, 73
mindful eating 73
miscarriage 3, 105, 132, 150, 157, 158, 160
misogyny 70, 139, 166, 209, 250
Moalem, Sharon 152
models, plus-sized 71
Mondelēz International 44, 80
monosodium glutamate (MSG) 153–4, 195, 271
Monteiro, Carlos 18, 33, 39–43, 172
mood 94, 134, 151, 175–6, 182–3, 195
Mosconi, Lisa 205–6
Moss, Kate 71
mother archetype 62, 64, 230
Mother Earth 229–31, 248
Mother Nature 229–31, 245, 247, 248, 306

mothers
  UPFs exploitation of 75–96
  see also maternal...
mouth bacteria (oral microbiome) 132, 174, 207
mouth feel 31
Mr Kipling 28, 113
Mrs. Butterworth 66–7
multinational food companies 4–5, 17, 44, 49, 95
multiple sclerosis (MS) 120, 154
mum-guilt 6
mustard 289
mycobiome 125

nappies 221
National Health Service (NHS) 129, 145, 150, 296
National School Lunch Program 115
Native American culture 10, 13, 229, 244
nature 9–10, 229–31, 244–5, 247–50, 306
Nestlé 44, 63, 69, 79–80, 82, 84–6, 88–9, 112, 232, 239, 307
Neubauer, Paula 236–7, 240
neuroinflammation 174
Neurology (journal) 206, 207
Newby, Karen 197
Nicoya, Costa Rica 208
nitrites/nitrates 296
'no added sugar' products 71

Nolan, Róisín 245–6
non-communicable diseases 39, 93
  see also chronic disease
non-stick coatings 219
noodles 21, 31
Norman, Noah Philip 37
Nova classification 18–23, 20, 33, 39, 43, 79, 104, 106, 172, 256, 290, 293, 299
NUTRIMUM trial 171
NutriNet-Santé 172
nutritional content 40
nutritional supplements 171, 177
nuts, flavoured 30

obesity 3, 5, 39–41, 43, 47, 53, 74, 97–116, 239
  and ageing 209
  and caesarean delivery 122
  definition 99
  as epidemic 99
  and fertility 149
  impact on women's health 105–7
  and insulin resistance 195
  and menarche 143
  and the menopause 195–6, 198
  and pregnancy 157–8, 160
  rise of 98–9, 108
  statistics 98–9
  and the vagina 156–7

vicious-cycle model of
    180–3, 184
obesity surgery (bariatric
    surgery) 112
oestrobolome 124, 126, 146,
    199
oestrogen 105–6, 124–6, 128,
    130, 142, 146, 223
    and body fat distribution
        194
    and dementia 205
    high levels of 124, 145
    and the menopause 187–8,
        196, 198–9
    see also phytoestrogens
Office for National Statistics
    (ONS) 73
oils 19, 290–3
olive oil 292, 293
Oliver, Catherine 147
omega-3 fatty acids 94, 146,
    150, 176–8, 184, 291–3
omega-6 fatty acids 291–3
'One Stone Solution' 112
Open Food Facts app 255, 257,
    289
Orang Rimba people 234
orangutans 233
organic produce 227, 249–50,
    255–6, 295, 299
Organisation for Economic Co-
    operation and Development
    (OECD) 99
orthorexia 72
osteoporosis 202–4

ovarian cancer 105, 106
overweight 93, 97, 104, 108
    and gallbladder problems
        200–1
    and pregnancy 157–8, 160
    statistics 98–9
    see also obesity
ovulation 105, 145, 150
Oxfam 235
oxidative stress 160, 170, 222
Ozempic 71, 112, 182

packaging 16, 17, 30, 41, 45,
    48, 50, 69, 71, 74, 83, 86, 95,
    102, 110, 207, 212–13, 214,
    218, 220, 222–4, 231–3, 239,
    248
    reusable/recyclable 226
packed lunches 92, 114–15,
    272–3
Palaeolithic era 142
palm oil 21–2, 27, 31–2, 48, 81,
    219, 233–5, 248, 271, 274,
    276, 279
pancake syrup 66–7
pancakes 66, 264, 297
parabens 224–5
Parkinson's 133
pasta 31
    pizza pasta (recipe) 284–5
patriarchy 13, 61, 74, 167,
    230–1, 307
Pearl Milling Company 66
people of colour 66–8, 222
pepperoni 285, 295–6

PepsiCo 44, 66, 68, 69, 78, 232
peptide YY (PYY) 41
per- and polyfluoroalkyl substances (PFAS) 219–21, 222
Percival, Rob 249–50
perfluorooctane sulfonic acid (PFOS) 220
periconceptional period 158
perimenopause 3, 130, 187–8, 192, 194, 197, 199
Philip Morris 44, 101–2, 232
phthalates 158–9, 221–2, 223
phytoestrogens 187–8, 189, 198, 205–6
pickles 135–6
pizza (recipe) 282–4
pizza pasta (recipe) 284–5
plant-based diets 89, 103, 187, 198, 208, 294–5
plant-based milks 254, 295
Plastic Soup app 218–19
plastics 10, 11, 16, 142, 149, 158–9, 207, 218–19, 222–3, 224, 227, 231–2, 247–8
pleasure of food 76–7
plus-sized models 71
Pollan, Michael 16, 187
polycystic ovary syndrome (PCOS) 105, 127–8, 147–8, 150, 161, 195, 222
popcorn 30, 96
postbiotics 137
potato wedges, homemade 287–8

Pratt, Lynne 200–1
pre-diabetes 194
pre-eclampsia 105, 132, 157, 158, 160
pre-menstrual syndrome (PMS) 43, 146–7, 179
pre-term birth 3, 126, 159–60, 221
prebiotics 103, 121, 133–4, 137, 199
pregnancy 2, 3, 43, 155–61, 213, 222
    and BPA 223, 224
    complications 105
    and geophagy 243
    and mental health 171, 178
    and the microbiome 130, 131–3
    and obesity 157–8
Premenstrual Dysphoric Disorder (PMDD) 179
preservatives 24
Price, Katie 72
Pringles 22, 41–2, 95, 208, 216
probiotics 134, 136–7, 143, 198, 200, 236
processed culinary ingredients 19, *20*
processed foods 18–23, *20*, 24, 31, 79, 290
    alcoholic beverages 33
    breakfasts 262
    highly processed 37, 38
    minimally processed 19, *20*, 26, 38, 206, 256

Nova 3 classification 19, 20, 24, 256
processed culinary ingredients 19, 20
see also ultra-processed foods
Procter & Gamble 216
profit-focus 4, 17, 25, 44–5, 84–90, 247, 307
progesterone 130, 145
prospective studies 172
prostaglandin 145
protein 5, 41, 150, 198
psychoanalytic theory 65
psychobiotics 175–6
puberty, onset in girls 141–4
public health crisis 44
pulses 31
Pyramid of Change 248, 249, 251

Quaker 66
Quince, Dawn 244–5

R. J. Reynolds 102
radio advertising 67–8
randomized controlled trials 40
rat studies 181–2, 202–3
ready-meals 281
Real Bread Campaign 28
recipes
    basic cookies 276
    broccoli and white bean soup 270
    the Dumas dressing 289–90
    easy crackers 267
    easy hummus 266
    easy mayo 288–9
    homemade potato wedges 287–8
    homemade stock 272
    pancakes 264
    pizza 282–4
    pizza pasta 284–5
    simple cupcakes 274–5
    spicy bean soup 269–70
    wraps 280
recycling 231–2
resilience 129
rheumatoid arthritis 154
rice 31
Ristorante 50
Romans 166
Rorty, James 37
Rose, Marcelle 72–3
rosemary extract 4
Rutt, Chris 66

Sainsbury's 80
salami 295–6
salt 19, 27, 40–2, 100–1, 147, 170, 195, 207, 261
Sardinia 208
sauces, tomato-based 281–2
saucisson 295–6
sauerkraut 135, 136–7
sausages 190, 296
schizophrenia 174, 183
Schlosser, Eric 215

school dinners 92, 114–15, 272–3
Scientific Advisory Committee on Nutrition (SACN) 79–80
sedentary lifestyles 100
seed oils 290–3
seeds 267
self-care 196
self-esteem, low 98, 107
self-harm 129, 173
self-service checkouts 11
self-sufficiency 246
serotonin 170, 173
sex 107, 166–8
sex chromosomes 151–2, 177, 212–13
sex differences 99, 108–9, 117–38, 175, 199
Sex Discrimination Act 1975 61
shakshuka 263, 264
shame 139–40
Shames, Laurence 39
shelf life 24–5, 45
short chain fatty acids 121, 133, 173–4
single-ingredient foods 257–8
Sjogren's syndrome 151
'skinny' products 71–2
slavery 66, 67
sleep apnea 105
sleep deprivation 183, 196
sleep problems 43, 183, 205
SlimFast 112, 113
smell, sense of 213, 214–15
SMILEs trial 172

smoking 44, 65, 103, 106, 110, 113–16, 158, 179–80, 203, 209
snacks
    ultra-processed 29–31, 45, 92, 146, 301
    UPF-free 265–7
social connection 10, 13
social disconnectedness 9, 11, 12, 74
soil 240–8
    eating (geophagy) 243
    erosion 240, 241, 243, 245
    microbes 242–3, 246
Solomon, Steve 246
soup 268–70
    broccoli and white bean 270
    spicy bean 269–70
    tinned 31
sourdough 28, 277–9
sourfaux 278
soy foods 149, 219, 235–9, 248, 295
Spare Rib (magazine) 61
sperm 3, 148–9
spirits 33, 34, 299
sponsors 78–80, 88–9, 114
spreads 293, 294
squashes 34
Standard American Diet (SAD) 169–73, 177, 187
Stevens, Nettie 151–2
Stevenson, Richard 180, 182
stigma, and body weight 98, 107

stock, homemade 272
stock cubes 271
stress 183–4, 196
suffering, women's 139–61, 185, 187, 189–90
sugar 19, 46, 86, 248
   see also 'low sugar' diets; 'no added sugar' products
sugar beet 241
sugary drinks 93, 143, 147, 160, 183, 190, 198
sugary foods 40–2, 69, 91, 100–1, 261, 297
   see also high sugar diets/foods
suicide 107, 129, 169, 173
supermarkets 10–11, 21, 24, 25–34, 47–8, 51, 278–9
Swan, Shanna 223–4
sweets 92, 93
Symbiotic Culture of Bacteria and Yeast (SCOBY) 134–5
Symrise 215

takeaways 95–6, 299–300
taste, sense of 213, 214–15
Tate & Lyle 69, 80
Teflon 219
telomeres 209
Tesco 21, 29
testosterone 194
Thanksgiving 10
thinness 71, 107
thrush 125
TikTok 68

tinned foods 31
titanium dioxide 217
tobacco companies 44, 65, 95, 101–2, 113–16
tomato 269–70, 283–5
   sauce 281–2
   tinned 281–2
'total diet' approach 78
'trad wives' 62
trans fats 70–1, 127, 150, 233
transglutaminase (meat glue) 95, 154–5
TV advertising 68
TV dinners 37–8

UK Biobank 2106
ultra-processed food (UPF) 1–13, 303–8
   addiction to 98, 110–11, 113, 116, 182–3, 193, 256
   and bone health 202–3
   carb to fat ratio 109, *109*
   characteristics 17
   contemporary debates surrounding 39–42
   and cosmetics 211, 215–20
   costs of 49–50
   craving 98, 102, 193, 197
   definition 15–35, 211, 255–7
   and dementia/cognitive decline 204, 206–7
   denigration of cooking skills 7, 12–13, 51, 57, 59–60, 63–4, 74, 307

and depression 169–75
and diabetes 195
distinction from processed foods 18–23
dog food 303–4, 307–8
eating more than you need of 17, 41–2, 100–2, 108–10
as 'edible foodlike substance' 16
environmental impact 230–41, 243–4, 247–8
evidence against 40–3
exploitation of mothers and children 75–96
food matrix 45–7, 102, 110, 121, 298
and gallbladder problems 200–2
grey areas 25
high-end/expensive 24
identification 255–7
and insomnia 18
and junk food 24–5
and the menopause 193, 195–8, 200
and the microbiome 117–38, 118–23
as misnomer 16–17
normalization 90, 93
not sweating the small stuff 257, 271, 277, 301–2
Nova 4 classification 20, *20*, 21–3, 24, 33, 256, 299
the problem with 37–57
as a product you were never meant to eat 34–5
profit-focus 4, 17, 25, 44–5, 84–90, 97, 247, 307
reason it is made 44–5
resistance to 13, 38, 43–4, 49–52, 77, 115–16
shelf life 24–5, 45
and telomere length 209
texture 24–5, 41, 100–1
and traditional gender roles 59–74
UPF swaps 248, **251**, 253–302
weight-loss claims 113
and women's suffering 139–61
women's toxic relationship with 97–116
see also packaging
ultra-processed food use disorder 110–11
ultra-processed products (UPPs) 16
Uncle Ben's rice (now Ben's Rice) 67
Underwood, Charles G. 66
Unilever 44, 78, 80, 215–16, 233
United Nations Environment Programme 232
unprocessed foods 19, *20*, 40, 206
Urinary Tract Infections (UTIs) 127

uterus 3
Utopian approach 249, **251**

vagina 156–7
vaginal fluids 121–3
vaginal microbiome 121–7, 137, 150, 161
van Tulleken, Chris 5, 16, 239
vapes 113
variety, dietary 53–5
vegan products 294–5
vegetables 26, 31
   see also specific vegetables
vicious cycles 169, 179–84
virtuous cycles 184
vitamin D 128, 149, 202, 204
Vogue magazine 71

Wade, Matt 244–5
Wainwright, Hannah 147–8
waist circumference 93, 195
Walkers 30
Wall Street (1987) 8
Wall Street Journal 115
Washington Post (newspaper) 68–9
water supplies (drinking) 220–1
weaning 62, 76, 78, 82, 90–1
   baby-led 91
Wegovy 71, 112, 182
weight 13, 98, 107, 191–4
   see also obesity; overweight
weight gain 100–1, 107
   abdominal 194
   and the dieting cycle 112–13

   and the menopause 192–4, 197
   and UPFs 40–1, 192–4
weight loss 104
   and dieting 112–15
   and the menopause 192, 193–4, 196
   unsuccessful 107, 108
   and willpower 193
weight training 188
weight-loss drugs 71, 112–13, 182
Western diet 38, 153, 154, 171, 182, 187, 207, 291
wholefoods 47, 56, 125, 146, 147, 248, 301
wild foods 54–6
Wildbiome™ Project 54–5
Wilde, Monica 54–5, 56
Wilson, Bee 16
wine 33, 299
Winnicott, Donald 76
witches 166–7
Wolf, Naomi 112
woman-blaming culture 156
womb cancer 105, 106
women 1–9, 12–13, 49, 57, 234–5, 237–9, 244–5, 250–1, 306–7
   'a woman's place' 59–74
   and ageing 185–210
   and bone health 202–4
   and cooking 6–7, 12–13
   as defective 166–7

and the double standards of
  ageing 209–10
eating patterns 108
and gall bladder problems
  200–2
labour 230
liberation from domestic
  drudgery 7, 12, 38, 74
medicalization 140
and mental health 165–72,
  175–6, 182–4
and the microbiome 117–38
and obesity 99
reduced to their
  reproductive potential 3
as sex class 231
and smoking 65
suffering of 139–61, 185,
  187, 189–90
toxic relationship with UPFs
  97–116
as UPF puppets 69
working 73–4

working hours 74
working women 73–4
World Health Organization
  (WHO) 68, 93–5, 171, 241
  the WHO Code 85, 90
World Obesity Federation 98
World Wildlife Fund (WWF)
  235, 238
wraps (recipe) 280

xanthan gum 32, 74, 121, 216,
  289

yoghurt 27, 143, 273, 294, 297
  ultra-processed 23–4, 27,
    70, 137
Yorkie bars 69
YouGov 73

ZOE personalised nutrition
  191, 195–6